EVERYTHING ABOUT SANKALPA YOGA

THE BIG BOOK ON CLASSICAL YOGA, DEEP RELAXATION & MEDITATION FOR CHAIR

Shreyanada Natha

Cover & Design
Mattias Långström

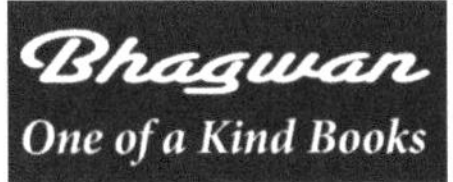

Everything about Sankalpa Yoga

THE BIG BOOK ON CLASSICAL YOGA, DEEP RELAXATION & MEDITATION FOR CHAIR

Shreyanada Natha

ISBN 9789198915419

✳✳✳

2 FREE BONUSES!

#1. Sign up for a **FREE TRIAL** *chair yoga class at the back of the book!*

#2. Download **CHAKRA-INDEX IN COLOR** *here!*

SCAN QR-CODE or go to:

https://bit.ly/47wdFVZ

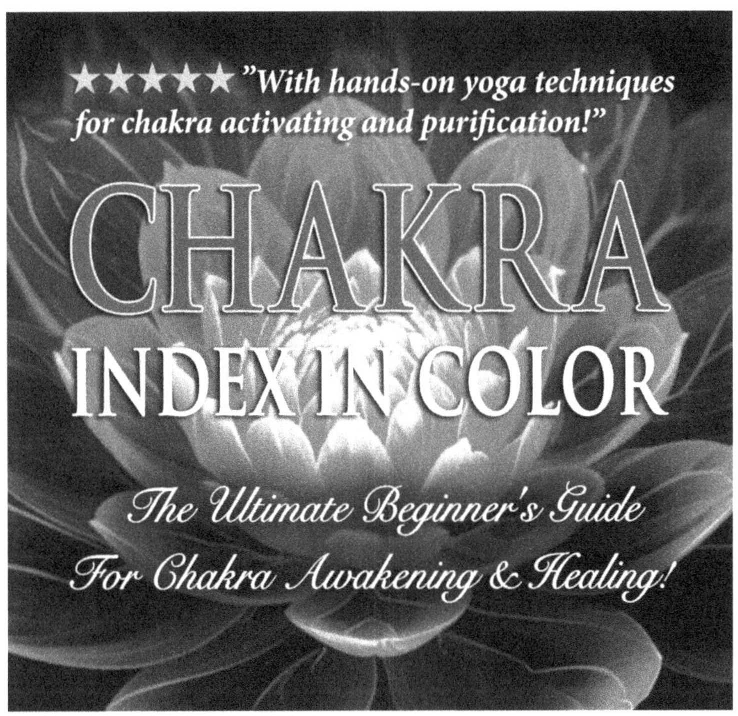

ABOUT THE BOOK

Sankalpa is a Sanskrit word – a deeply rooted intention or desire. In the Patanjali Yoga Sutras, the first verse is Atha Yoga Anushasanam, which means that the learning of yoga is now starting, that yoga is here and now, and that it is never too late to start or continue. In Sankalpa yoga, the practitioner takes a stand for their well-being by performing classical chair yoga decisively and purposefully to promote their health and flexibility despite physical limitations.

MY NAME AND MY MISSION

Shreyananda Natha was the name I received when I was initiated into the Natha Order and received the master mantra—Shodasi-mantra—after studying yoga and tantra for over twelve years. Shodasi-mantra is the highest mantra in yoga and tantra. It means "he who knows."

After practicing yoga and meditation continuously for over 20 years, having a yoga school for many years, and leading studies for yoga teachers, I wanted to reach out more broadly with yoga, out into our whole society, out of the little yoga room. Spread the knowledge of yoga, our chakra system, and Kundalini Shakti to everyone who wants to listen. What needed to be added were sensible factual books on yoga that were in-depth educational and not just skim the surface or were about the author's private life. So it became my Sankalpa, my magical wish, and my mission to create exciting yoga books that everyone can read and enjoy. To show how we can apply and use yoga in different parts of life and achieve success and health. Here and now.

So, if you like my books, please follow me on my social media, share and like them, tell your friends about them, and write an honest review; one or two lines don't matter. All support is precious.

MY YOUTUBE CHANNEL

My YouTube channel, **YOGA BEYOND THE POSES***, has been a significant project for me. I wanted to create a channel containing my two most extensive life interests: yoga, of course, and everything related to the mystery of life, the spiritual and the psychic. Yes, everything related to the expansion of our consciousness. What we experience in yoga beyond the poses…*

I broadcast LIVE on YouTube, and during the broadcast, I talk about yoga and spirituality and let viewers ask questions that I answer with the help of runes and what I receive as a medium. It's completely free, and it would be great to hear your question and see what the runes say about it. You can subscribe to the channel to quickly get notifications before each broadcast so you don't miss any exciting questions.

Scan the QR code or visit:
https://shorturl.at/dqx36

THE AUTHOR

Shreyananda Natha is the author of popular and best-selling yoga books. He has written one of the most comprehensive books on yoga – EVERYTHING ABOUT YOGA and the study book – TEACHING YOGA AND MEDITATION BEYOND THE PO-SES. He is also a certified yoga & meditation teacher according to the international guidelines of EYTF. He has undergone several years of yoga teacher training under the guidance of Swami Omananda at Satyananda Ashram and holds the highest initiation in the tantric Natha order. He frequently travels to Asia and India to deepen his knowledge and gather inspiration. He has immersed himself in tantric rituals and is known for his extensive knowledge of yoga, deep relaxation, and meditation.

"There is no authority that can say what yoga is. When you give yourself completely and thoroughly and experience yoga without limitations and doubts, the actual meeting with yoga arises when you become one with the experience within you. Only then do you understand what yoga is – for you. When you are no longer limited by modesty, shyness, and artificial thought patterns that act as a filter between you and trans-formation.

Yoga is a cultural richness still passed on from teacher to student and helps man find his true nature. It opens us up and attracts awareness. It strengthens our self-esteem, and our entire spectrum of possibilities suddenly becomes visible. Yoga is easy and normal. You don't need to become vegan, a monk, or be able to stand on your head. You need to do your yoga regularly; the rest will come naturally. You can use yoga and meditation to feel better physically and mentally and succeed and develop in all areas of life – here and now.

Good luck!"

Namasté

I want to thank the teachers and students I have had over the years who have made my journey with yoga so enjoyable. Thank you for all the inspiration you have given me and for making this book possible. The yoga masters who no longer live among us – live on with each new person who delves into the yoga tradition.

Sri Swami Sivananda, Sri Swami Satyananda, Sri Tirumalai Krishnamacharya, Sri Swami Vishnudevananda, Sri K. Pattabhi Jois, Osho, Swami Nirdosha, Swami Omananda, Swami Janakananda, Ole Schmidt, Turiya, Maryam Abrishami, and Sanna Kuittinen.

All the people who have sought answers to what they have sensed through an activated Ajna chakra. In yoga, they have learned the principles behind the universe, the collective consciousness, and the creative power, Kundalini Shakti. The duality behind everything, both what we see and what we don't see. Together, we help pass on the previously secret knowledge about our gunas, nadis, and chakras to everyone who wants to be a Rishi.

Aum Shri Durgayai Namaha

INDEX

MEDICAL DISCLAIMER

A doctor should always be consulted before practicing yoga in case of any injury or illness. It should never hurt joints, complex parts, or ligaments during execution. Inverted asanas should be avoided in cases of gas formation, late pregnancy, and menstruation. One should never sunbathe immediately after yoga due to the risk of overheating.

1

INTRODUCTION

WHAT DOES RESEARCH SAY ABOUT THE HEALTH BENEFITS OF YOGA?

Yoga has become increasingly popular worldwide as a holistic exercise method that promotes physical, mental, and emotional well-being. Research has explored the many benefits of regularly practicing yoga, and a wide range of health benefits have been found. These range from improved flexibility and strength to reduced stress and anxiety.

One of yoga's most apparent physical benefits is improved flexibility and mobility. By performing various yoga exercises that stretch and strengthen the muscles, practitioners can achieve increased flexibility in the body. A study published in the Journal of Bodywork and Movement Therapies found that a 12-week yoga program significantly improved participants' flexibility compared to a control group that did not engage in yoga (Williams et al., 2005).

In addition to increased flexibility, yoga has improved strength and muscle tone. Yoga practitioners strengthen different muscle groups throughout the body by performing various positions and postures that require balance and stability. A study published in the Journal of Strength and Conditioning Research found that an eight-week yoga program significantly improved muscle strength and endurance among participants (Tran et al., 2016).

In addition to its physical benefits, yoga has been shown to positively affect mental and emotional health. Many people use yoga to manage stress and anxiety and promote relaxation and calmness. A review article published in the Harvard Health Blog summarizes several studies showing that yoga can reduce stress hormones and promote relaxation in the nervous system (Harvard Health Publishing, 2018).

In addition to reducing stress, yoga has been shown to affect mental clarity and cognitive function positively. A study published in the Journal of Physical Activity and Health found that participants who regularly practiced yoga had better cognitive performance and faster reaction times than non-practicing control groups (Gothe et al., 2013).

In summary, research suggests that yoga can be a versatile exercise method that promotes physical health by increasing flexibility and strength and contributes to mental well-being by reducing stress and promoting relaxation and cognitive clarity. Considering these many health benefits, it's no wonder that yoga has become so popular as a holistic health practice worldwide.

WHAT IS YOGA?

Classical Indian yoga, as described in the Patanjali Yoga Sutras, is a concept developed to bring people into balance in everything. Balance in our actions, our physical body and breath, our energy body (prana in our nadis), our doshas, yes, everything to gradually quiet the mind and, through focused attention, attain deep insights and bring about a natural expansion of consciousness through meditation. Patanjali described it as the eightfold path. From ethics and morality to asanas (yoga postures), breathing exercises (pranayamas), and beyond from the body to the mind and meditation. A progression from the gross to the subtle and purest. From movement to absolute stillness. In body and mind.

Hatha yoga is yoga on the way, which involves using your body to prepare the mind for meditation. Yes, what you do with your physical body gradually balances the mind. Hatha yoga contains five components or parts: purification exercises (shatkarmas), body positions (asanas), breathing exercises (pranayamas), mudras (postures), and bandhas (locks).

CAN YOU PRACTICE YOGA ON A CHAIR?

When I developed my concept of classical chair yoga, I wanted to open the door for everyone to find a way into yoga, from those who attend yoga classes in studios a few times a week to those who have never tried yoga for various reasons, and for all the people out there with different forms of physical and mental obstacles.

Yoga for all ages and all needs. Yes, it is a form of yoga that can be practiced daily at home or elsewhere, independent of studios, mats, and obstacles. But I had one requirement: it must be a real, genuine classical yoga in its proper context. Not some expressed yoga-inspired exercises on a chair. No, the experience of my chair yoga would be just as absolute as attending an advanced classical yoga class. It would contain all the parts and components, from Hatha yoga to yogic deep relaxation and meditation.

When I looked around, I found several books on chair yoga, but they all showed the same thing – yoga-inspired movements on a chair. Not classical yoga for a chair. I thought about Patanjali's description of asanas and the meaning of the word yoga – yoga chitta vritti nirodha (to still the mind). I understood what I wanted to create. I also understood that I couldn't call my concept "chair yoga." It would just make people think it was a yoga-inspired exercise. No, I had to have a name so people grasp the concept but still understand that it is connected to a chair. But what on earth should I call the yoga? If I did this wrong, I understood that no one would understand the concept, or it would be misinterpreted. The name was necessary. Important. After thinking long and hard, I eventually settled on the name. No matter how I twisted and turned the concept, I always ended up with the practitioner's decision and desire with their yoga: to achieve a better life on various levels. A desire for something better ... regardless.

Sankalpa is a Sanskrit word meaning – a deeply rooted intention or desire. It symbolizes a robust inner desire or decision. In the context of chair yoga, Sankalpa yoga can convey that through this style of yoga, one can create a strong inner intention or desire for better health and well-being despite any physical limitations. In the Patanjali Yoga Sutras, the first verse is Atha Yoga Anushasanam, which means that the learning of yoga is now starting, that yoga is here and now, and it's never too late to start or to continue.

Yes, the practitioner takes a stand for their own well-being by performing yoga positions with the help of a chair decisively and purposefully to promote their own health and flexibility: Sankalpa yoga—classical yoga for a chair. The name was born: yoga, deep relaxation, and meditation for a chair.

My second challenge was creating the flow of yoga to have my desired effect. I would only succeed if I showed the positions in pictures in a book with instructions. I had to convey the rhythm, the feeling, and the deep relaxation/meditation. Otherwise, I knew I wouldn't at least succeed in conveying the

experience of a genuinely genuine classical yoga class. I un-
derstood I had to guide the participants through the sequences
and lead the meditations. A book is excellent in every way, but
the voice must be there. I decided to create my yoga channel
on YouTube. I also understood that the participants would
gradually develop a greater interest in personal development
and a deepened interest in the spiritual and mystical aspects
of existence through Sankalpa yoga. Yes, all that we experi-
ence beyond the poses in yoga.

My YouTube channel was Yoga Beyond the Poses, which in-
cludes my most significant life interests. The classical, genuine
yoga and everything around the spiritual. I also have a keen
interest in rune reading and have long helped people as a
medium/psychic with questions about everything they expe-
rience as most important in life.

I started with the spiritual and then worked intensively with
the yoga, filming all the positions and assembling powerful
sequences and series matching the participants' sankalpas:
desires for results. So please look at some episodes if you have
the time and inclination; they cost nothing: **YouTube @yo-**
gabeyondtheposes.

MORE ABOUT YOGA

In Patanjali's Yoga Sutras, there is a definition of asanas —
Stirham Sukham Asana, which means steady/comfortable

posture. The aim was to develop the ability to sit still for a more extended period, which was a prerequisite for meditation.

However, within Hatha yoga, it was discovered that certain specific positions, asanas, opened up energy channels and psychic centers in the body. This provided better body control and, thereby, the ability to develop control over thoughts, the mind, and energies. Yoga asanas became a tool to achieve higher consciousness and provided a stable foundation to explore the body, breath, and mind.

Initially, there were eight million four hundred thousand different asanas. These represent as many lives as an unenlightened person must be reborn before enlightenment. Rishis and yogis narrowed down the number to a few hundred known today. From those, they selected the eighty-four most essential asanas. Thirty-five asanas directly impact our chakras. The rest purify and regulate our nadis (energy channels). Asanas create a balance between body and mind and a flow in the sushumna nadi (the energy channel along the spine that only opens when you are balanced).

Rishis studied animals and could see how they lived harmoniously with their bodies and surroundings. By mimicking animals' movement patterns and body positions, they could affect hormone secretion. During deep meditation, they could *observe how different body positions affected the body and the mind.*

The vital energy (life energy), prana, permeates our entire body. Poor flow of prana in the body results in stiffness and an accumulation of toxins. When prana can flow freely, these toxins are eliminated, and the body becomes soft and flexible. Even the most difficult positions become easy to perform. When the amount of prana increases in the body, one achieves "pranic intuition." One understands how asanas, mudras, and pranayamas should be performed intuitively.

Hatha yoga improves overall health and activates our energy centers by balancing the nervous system. Asanas in Hatha yoga also release tensions that arise as knots in our muscles. By releasing these tensions from the body, we also release tensions from the mind. It makes us feel better overall and releases underlying and latent energy.

So, asanas are not just exercises. They are techniques that place the body in different positions to promote awareness, relaxation, concentration, and meditation. Part of this process is developing a good physique through stretching, stimulating prana, and massaging glands and internal organs.

Asanas are divided into three groups: beginners, intermediate, and advanced. It is optional to perform all the exercises in each group. Daily practice of a tailored program for individual needs is optimal for achieving the most significant effect.

Beginner-level asanas should be performed by those who have never practiced yoga before. These have a more significant effect on beginners' bodies than advanced practitioners. These exercises prepare the body and mind for more advanced exercises and meditation, which help improve physical health.

Intermediate-level exercises are for those who can perform beginner-level exercises without difficulty. These require greater concentration, stability, and coordination in movement and breathing.

Advanced asanas are for those with well-developed body control, muscles, and nervous systems. One should be able to master the intermediate-level exercises without difficulty. It is essential to take your time and start these exercises early enough.

DYNAMIC AND STATIC ASANAS

Dynamic asanas increase flexibility and circulation in the body. They loosen muscles, release knots, and energy blockages, and remove stagnant blood. These asanas are most important for beginners. To work with, for example, the chakra system, one must first release blockages. Otherwise, energy can flow in the wrong direction in the energy body. The dynamic asanas and vinyasas process our physical body and take us deeper, preparing us for the more static asanas. Often, Hatha yoga begins with a lot of movement and then gradually allows the vibrations to settle into stillness and silence. It also has a lot to do with moving from the gross to the subtle – from the body to the mind– and understanding how yoga affects our doshas through Ayurveda.

VINYASA

Dynamic asanas are often synchronized with the breath. When we do this, it is called vinyasa. A flow where movements and breath work together.

The purpose of vinyasa is to increase internal purification and detoxification of the body. Breathing synchronized with movement heats the blood. Thick blood is often unhealthy and causes diseases. The heat from vinyasa purifies the blood and thins it so it can circulate better in the body, around our joints, and reduce pain. Where the body has poor circulation, pain usually arises. The heated blood also passes through all the internal organs, carrying away impurities and diseases that are removed from the body with increased sweat during the yoga session.

Sweat is an essential byproduct of vinyasa. It is only through our sweat that diseases can leave the body and be purified, in the same way that gold is melted to eliminate impurities.

Yoga boils the blood and transports impurities and toxins to the surface, which are subsequently removed with the help of sweat. If vinyasa is practiced frequently, the body becomes healthy, strong, pure, and shining like gold.

Once the body is purified, it is possible to purify the nervous system and sensory organs.

STATIC ASANAS

Static, especially inverted, asanas have the most profound effect on our energy body and chakra system. These require greater flexibility and are for more experienced practitioners. One remains in the position for a few minutes, which has a more powerful effect on glands, prana, chakras, and internal organs. The mind becomes calm and prepares the individual for meditation. Some static asanas are beneficial for reaching pratyahara (the first step in meditation).

TRISTHANA

Tristhana means three areas to focus on: posture (position, stretching, and relaxation), breath, and gaze point. They are always performed in conjunction with each other.

Asanas purify, strengthen, and soften the body. When we breathe with rechaka and puraka, with a steady and even inhalation and exhalation at the same pace, we purify the nervous system. You look at Drishti during yoga practice; there are nine different points: the nose, eyebrow center, navel, thumb, hands, feet, right and left side, and upward. Drishti purifies, captures, and stabilizes the mind.

ADVICE FOR PRACTICING ASANAS

BREATHING

According to Hatha Yoga, air and fire are two components that cleanse the body internally. Fire – our life force, is located at the solar plexus in the body and is generated by the Manipura chakra. For the fire to burn, air is required. Hence, it is essential to practice correct breathing in yoga. Even breaths increase the inner fire – agni in the body, which heats up the blood for physical purification and burns impurities in the nervous system. When the inner fire increases in strength, our digestive system, health, and lifespan also improve. Irregular breathing creates an imbalance in our physical body and signaling systems and impairs our immune system. According to Hatha yoga, we risk becoming ill in the long run – we have deteriorated protection and tolerance to both stress and toxins.

Another important component for increasing the inner fire is to use moola and uddiyana bandha, root and stomach locks. They increase the effectiveness of breathing, hold the energy inside the body longer, encapsulate it, and give light, strength, and health to the body.

According to Hatha yoga, six poisons in the body surround our spiritual heart. These poisons obscure the light in our hearts: desire, anger, delusion, greed, envy, and sloth. When we practice Hatha yoga for a long time with strength, determination, and proper breathing, the increasing heat in the body will burn up these six poisons, and the light in our inner self will shine through. We will feel better both mentally and emotionally.

It is important to breathe through the nose (unless otherwise stated) and coordinate the breathing with the movement. But never force yourself to breathe through the nose. If you need to breathe through the mouth, do so. Your fine energy channels can otherwise be damaged, and the energy can flow in the wrong direction in the energy body. If you become too breathless, wait for the breath until you can breathe through the nose again without it feeling too difficult.

AWARENESS

The purpose of asanas is to influence and create harmony in all aspects of the human being: physically, mentally, emotionally, pranic, and spiritually. By performing asanas consciously, all these parts are affected. One should be aware of bodily sensations, movement, and position, and in coordination with the breath, the flow of prana. One should focus on the chakras and witness thoughts and feelings that arise.

RELAXATION

One can lie down in shavasana at any time for rest or contemplation or sit still on a chair with a straight spine. Feel how it feels in the body and calm the breathing.

SEQUENCE

Always start with shatkarmas (cleansing processes), e.g., nasal rinsing/jala neti – then perform asanas, pranayamas, pratyahara, and dharana (concentration/quiet the mind) leading to dhyana (meditation). You can also incorporate both breathing exercises and meditation before asanas. It serves a purpose – especially at the beginning of your yoga practice, to start from the outside and move in before intuitively feeling what, when, and how to do it.

COUNTERPOSE

It is essential to have a structure in the program to balance the body and nervous system. A forward-bending position should always be followed by a backward-bending position and vice versa. So, a yoga program is carefully constructed by knowledgeable yogis and is not something you do haphazardly like regular warm-ups. However, this does not apply to yoga rehabilitation.

TIME

Asanas can be practiced at any time of the day, provided you have not eaten for 2–3 hours. However, practicing just before sunrise and just before sunset is recommended. The time of day just before sunrise is called Brahmamuhurta (the divine time – God's time). The atmosphere is then pure and still, the stomach and intestines inactive, and the mind calm. The most favorable time is before sunrise and then before sunset, but do not be too ambitious from the beginning. Having a yoga session at any time during the day is better than having none at all. Right?

PLACE

One should find a secluded place that is tidy, clean, calm, and quiet. You can also practice outdoors in a comfortable and beautiful place, not in cold and windy weather, where the air is polluted, or in glaring sun.

CHOICE OF CHAIR OR MAT

If using a chair, it is essential that it is stable and cannot slide or slip away. If we practice on a mat, use a mat made of natural material. It has the most favorable effect on our pranic streams. Choose a mat you can use for many years to come of the best quality; prana is stored in the mat and has a beneficial effect on the body. So, take care of your mat and cherish it tenderly. Make sure you can lie on it comfortably and that it is not too small or too thin so the surface is felt through if, for example, you stand on your head. It should be cushioning but still provide a good grip. A good mat lasts ten years or more, so do not be stingy with yourself. Treat yourself to a premium mat of the right size and feel.

CLOTHING

Wear loose and comfortable clothing, remove jewelry, and be barefoot so you do not slip if you practice on a mat. Prana is also stored in your yoga clothes.

SHOWER

Try to take a cold shower before the session to awaken the body. Wait to shower after the session so you do not unnecessarily cool down the body too quickly and lose the health benefits of yoga.

TOILET

Empty the stomach.

DIET

There are no strict rules for what food to eat. However, a natural diet in moderate amounts is recommended so that not all energy is used to digest food. A vegetarian diet is not essential but recommended. The stomach should be filled halfway with food, a quarter with water, and a quarter should be left empty. However, do not drink water during the session as it draws blood and energy to the stomach and cools down your energy body. After all, we want to get the power into the body during yoga, as is well known. Also, wait two to three hours after eating before yoga so that it does not feel uncomfortable and unpleasant during the session.

EXECUTION

Asanas are performed gently and carefully in three steps:

Awareness of the body, movement, and thoughts that arise. This creates calm, balance, and focus, leading to a state of harmony in the body. Feel that you do not tense up in the exercise.

Awareness of breathing. Synchronize movement with breathing. The movement becomes calmer, and brain waves become slower. You become relaxed and gain increased awareness.

Awareness of the flow of prana. You can experience it as tingling in the body. You develop the feeling through regular practice. You get mental calmness, become focused, and emotionally receptive.

Asanas are also divided into three parts:

Starting position.
Execution.
Final position.

IMPORTANT TO REMEMBER

A doctor should always be consulted before practicing yoga in case of any injury or illness. It should never hurt joints, complex parts, or ligaments during execution. Inverted asanas should be avoided in cases of gas formation, late pregnancy, and menstruation. One should never sunbathe immediately after yoga due to the risk of overheating.

REFERENCES

Williams, K., Abildso, C., Steinberg, L., Doyle, E., Epstein, B., Smith, D., ... & Cooper, L. (2005). Evaluation of the effectiveness and efficacy of Iyengar yoga therapy on chronic low back pain. Spine, 30(6), 660-666.

Tran, M. D., Holly, R. G., Lashbrook, J., Amsterdam, E. A., & Hanelin, J. (2001). Effects of Hatha yoga practice on the health related aspects of physical fitness. Preventive cardiology, 4(4), 165-170.

Harvard Health Publishing. (2018). Yoga for anxiety and depression. Harvard Health Blog. Hämtad från https://www.health.harvard.edu/mind-and-mood/yoga-for-anxiety-and-depression.

Gothe, N. P., McAuley, E., & Yoga, A. C. (2013). Yoga is as good as stretching–strengthening exercises in improving functional fitness outcomes: results from a randomized controlled trial. Journal of Physical Activity and Health, 10(3), 406-414.

2

WARM-UP

WARM-UP

Warm-up is vital before starting a yoga session and is essential for several reasons. By performing a warm-up routine before you begin your yoga poses, you prepare the body physically and mentally for the upcoming activity.

Prevents injuries: Warm-up helps prepare the muscles, tendons, and joints by gradually increasing blood flow. It reduces the risk of injuries during yoga by making the body more flexible and ready for movement.

Increases mobility: Dynamic stretching exercises and movements during warm-up improve the body's mobility and flexibility. They make it easier to perform yoga poses with correct form and reduce the risk of muscle strain.

Improves performance: Warming up increases the body's temperature and improves nerve-muscle coordination. It can lead to better execution of yoga poses and increased strength and endurance during the practice.

Mental focus: Warm-up also provides an opportunity to shift focus from everyday stress and distractions to the upcoming yoga practice. It can help create a mental space for presence and mindfulness during the workout.

Several physiological changes occur in the body during warm-up:

Increased blood flow: As the body warms up, blood flow to the muscles increases, improving oxygen and nutrient supply to the tissues and helping to eliminate waste products.

Increased body temperature: Warm-up increases the body's temperature, making the muscles more elastic and reducing the risk of injuries.

Activation of the nervous system: Warm-up movements activate the nervous system and improve nerve-muscle coordination, resulting in smoother and more efficient movements during yoga practice.

Improved joint mobility: By performing movements that stretch and move the joints, warm-up increases joint mobility and reduces stiffness.

By including a warm-up routine in your yoga practice, you can reduce the risk of injuries, improve mobility and performance, and increase mental focus during the workout.

INSTRUCTIONS BEFORE THE YOGA SESSION

Cleanse the nose with a neti pot (a nasal rinsing can with lukewarm water and salt) or nasal spray. Do not eat heavy food approximately 2-3 hours before. Preferably, be vegetarian. Do not drink caffeine. All of this calms the mind and gets the blood and prana moving in the body. Sit relaxed with a straight back.

START – MOUNTAIN POSE

One of the most commonly used positions is the mountain pose – the mountain, and although it is a neutral sitting position, it has various benefits. It is an essential position used in yoga to begin a pose or routine. It helps improve your posture and increases your awareness to discover other areas in your body that may be tense. It's an easy position to learn. It focuses the mind on yoga and centers you.

MOUNTAIN POSE

Sit in your chair with your feet hip-width apart and your hands resting on your thighs or knees. Inhale to engage your core muscles and lift your spine. As you exhale, imagine your body rooting itself to the ground and feel your sitting bones against the chair seat. Press all four corners of your feet onto the floor. Draw your shoulders down and back as you take a deep breath in. Hold for about a minute.

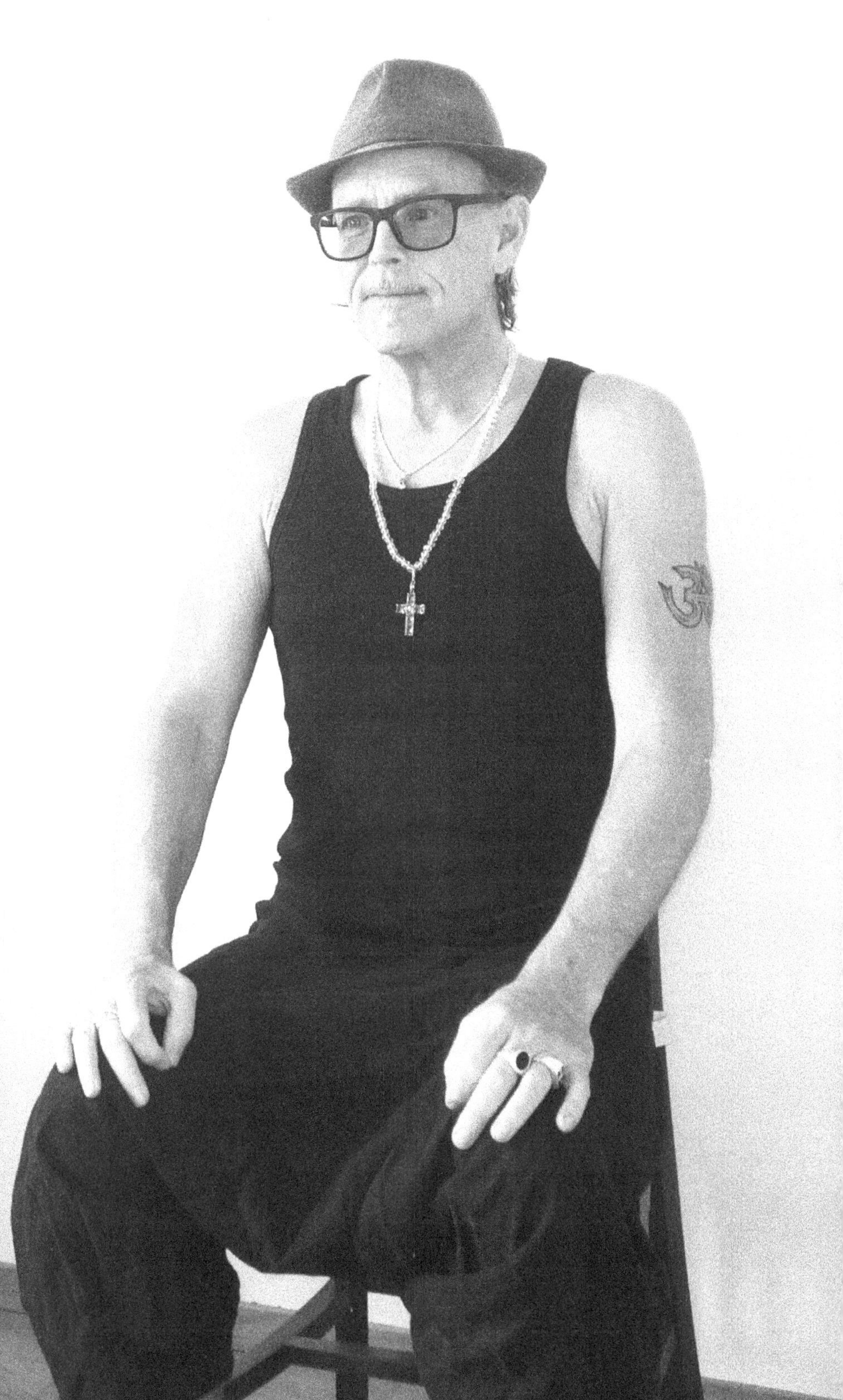

MOUNTAIN POSE WITH EXTENDED ARMS

Sit in your chair with your legs hip-width apart and your hands resting on your thighs or hanging by your sides. Inhale and lift your arms overhead. Join your fingers while keeping your index fingers and thumbs out so that you point directly toward the ceiling. Exhale and roll your shoulders away from your ears. Stay with your arms extended overhead for five breaths. Release and gently let your arms return to your sides.

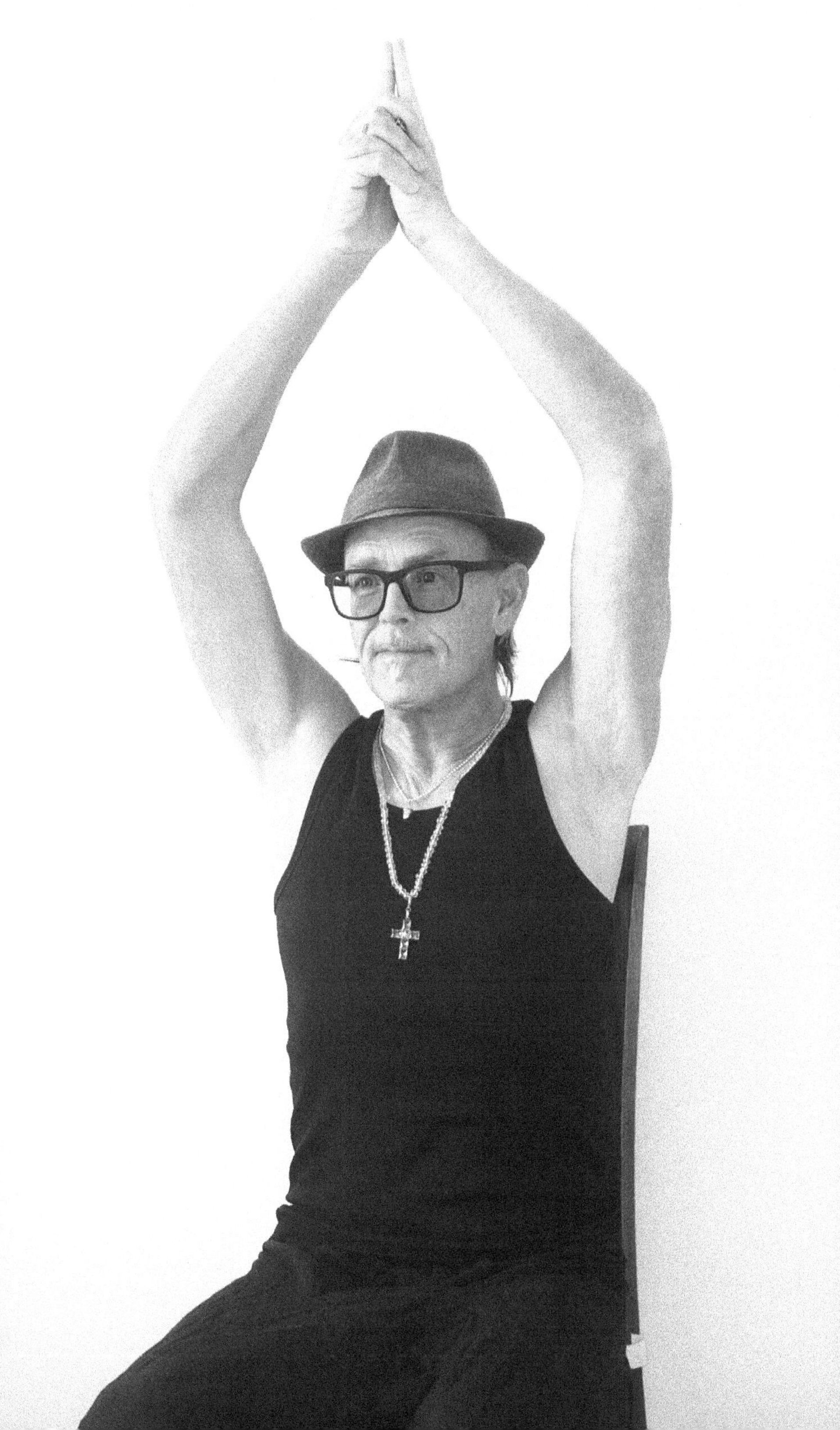

SUN SALUTATION

The Sun Salutation, also known as Surya Namaskara in Sans-krit, is traditionally used at the beginning of a yoga practice. It is an opportunity to open up all parts of the body before the yoga practice.

Start in a seated Mountain Pose (a neutral position) with your knees over your ankles, hip-width apart. Inhale, lift your arms overhead, reaching upward as if trying to touch the ceiling. Exhale into a prayer position as you bring your hands to your heart. Keeping the hands in the same position, fold forward and round your spine. Open your hands to reach the floor, letting them rest on your shins, ankles, or the floor. Inhale and roll up and arch (possibly looking up). Roll your shoulders so they draw away from your ears, and come back to Mountain Pose and relax.

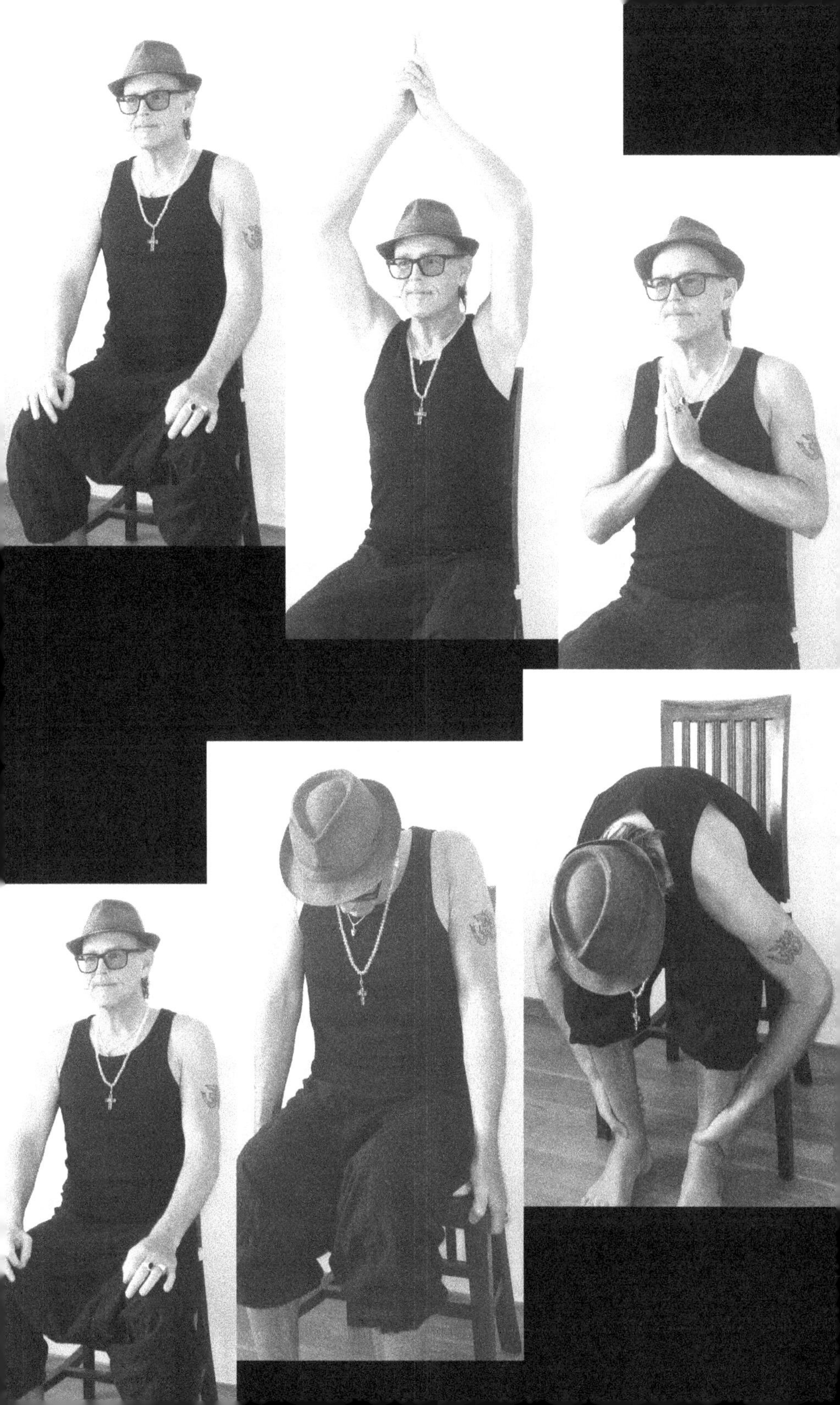

CAT

The Cat is a movement that involves moving your spine from a rounded position to an arched one in conjunction with your breath. By flexing and extending the spine through this movement, you allow circulation around your vertebrae to improve, release tension or pain in the lower back and spine, and improve your posture. The Cat also helps stretch your hips, abdomen, and chest muscles.

Start in a seated Mountain Pose with your knees over your ankles, hip-width apart. Place your hands on your knees. Inhale and look up at the ceiling. As you exhale, round your back, draw your navel towards your spine, and look down at your belly. Finish in the Mountain Pose.

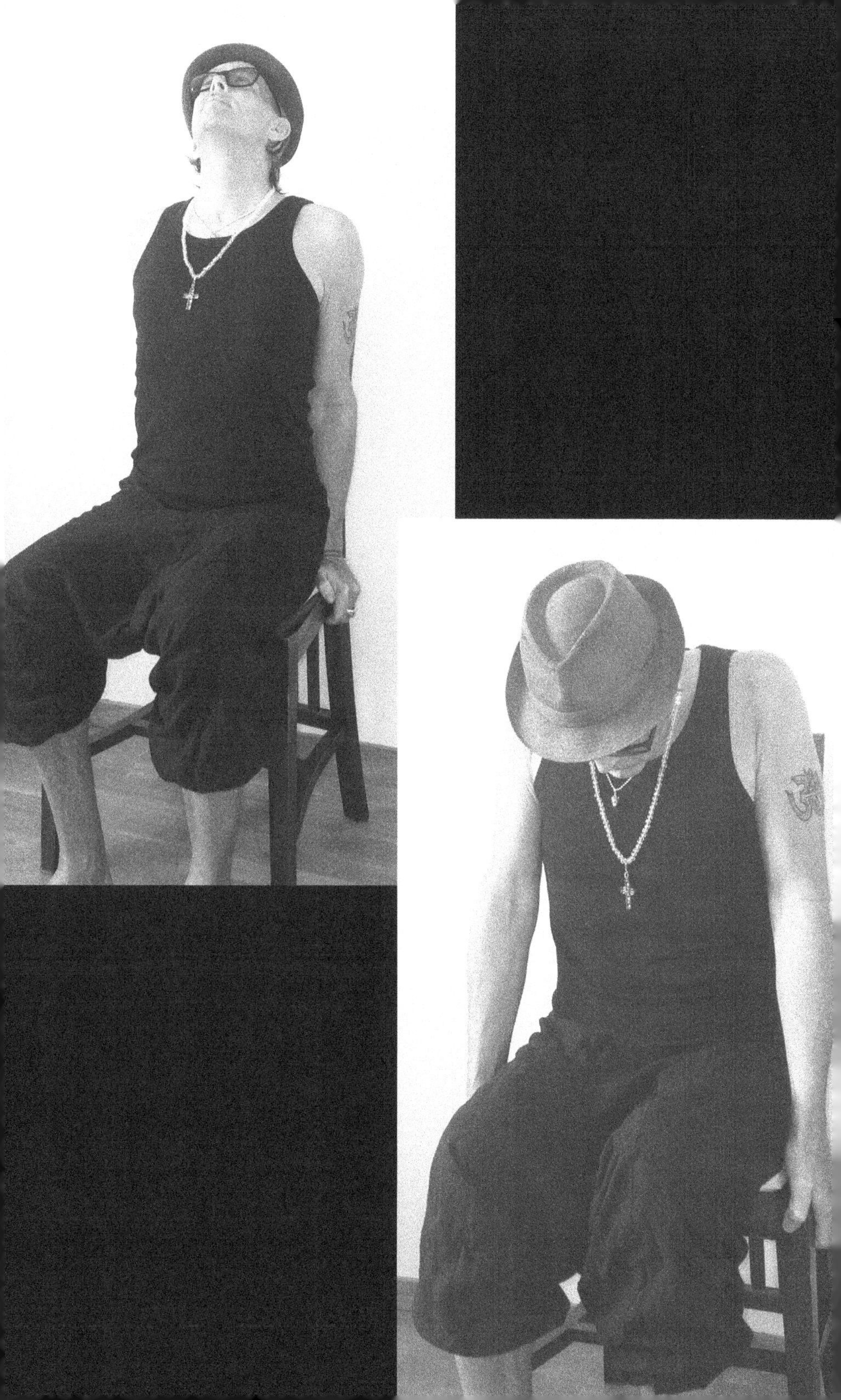

FORWARD BEND

Whether from a chair or standing, forward bends are an excellent way to stretch and lengthen your hamstrings and calves. This movement will also stretch your hips and lower back.

Start in a seated mountain pose with your knees over your ankles, hip-width apart. Place your hands on your thighs. As you inhale, lengthen your spine. Exhale and slowly bend forward. Extend your hands towards your feet or the floor. Let your head hang heavy to allow relaxation in the neck. Inhale and exhale, allowing your hamstrings and lower back to feel the stretch. When you're ready to sit up, inhale and slowly roll up, letting your head come up last. Finish in mountain pose.

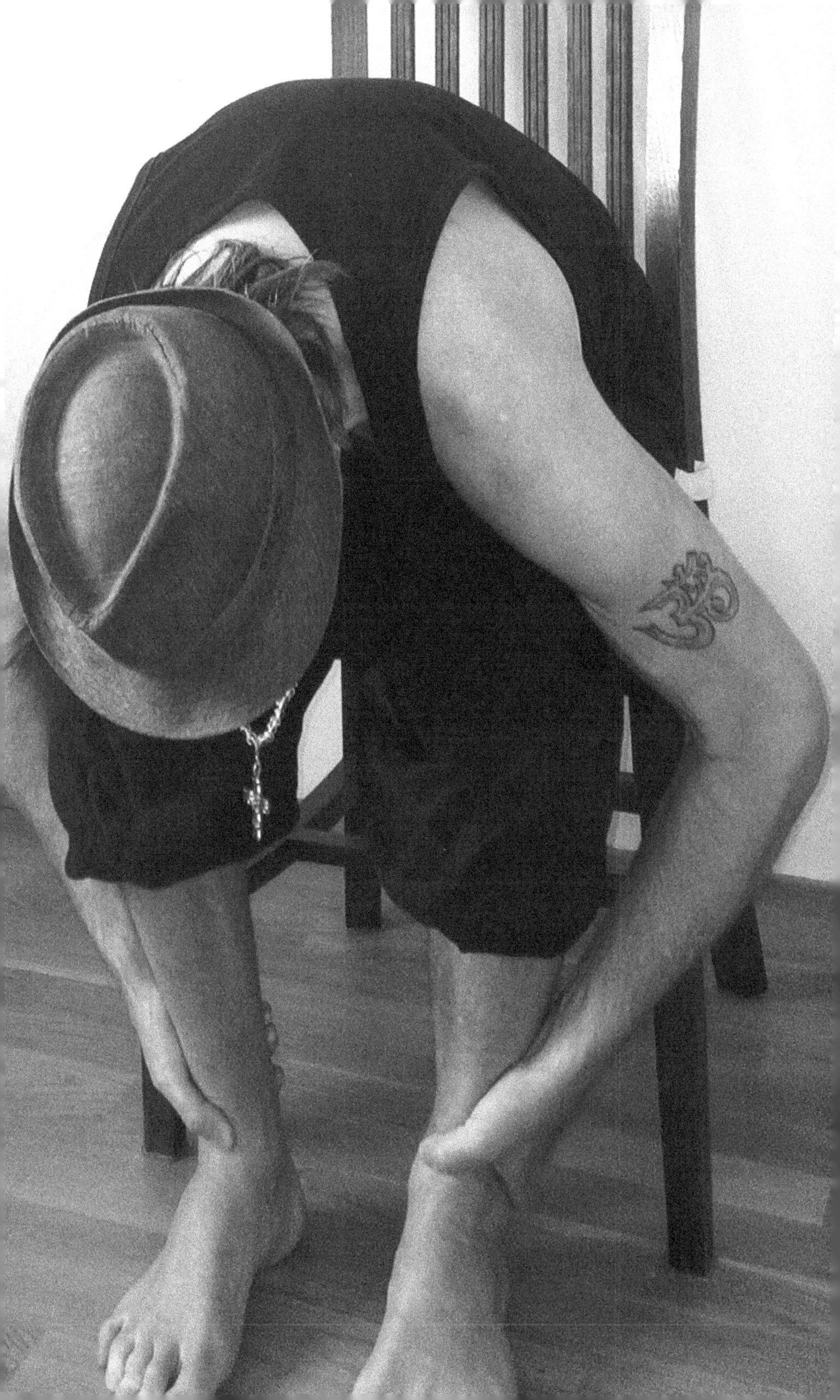

SIDE BEND

Side bends are an excellent way to stretch your side muscles and release any tension you may have there. The movements also open up your chest. Additionally, the side bending motion can increase mobility and flexibility, strengthen your core muscles, improve your posture, and enhance circulation.

Start in a seated mountain pose with your knees over your ankles, hip-width apart. Your arms hang by your sides. Inhale and lift your left arm overhead, palm facing inward. Place your right hand beside the chair for stability. Exhale as you bend towards your right side. Inhale and return to the starting position. Exhale and lower your left arm to repeat the same steps on the left side. Finish in mountain pose.

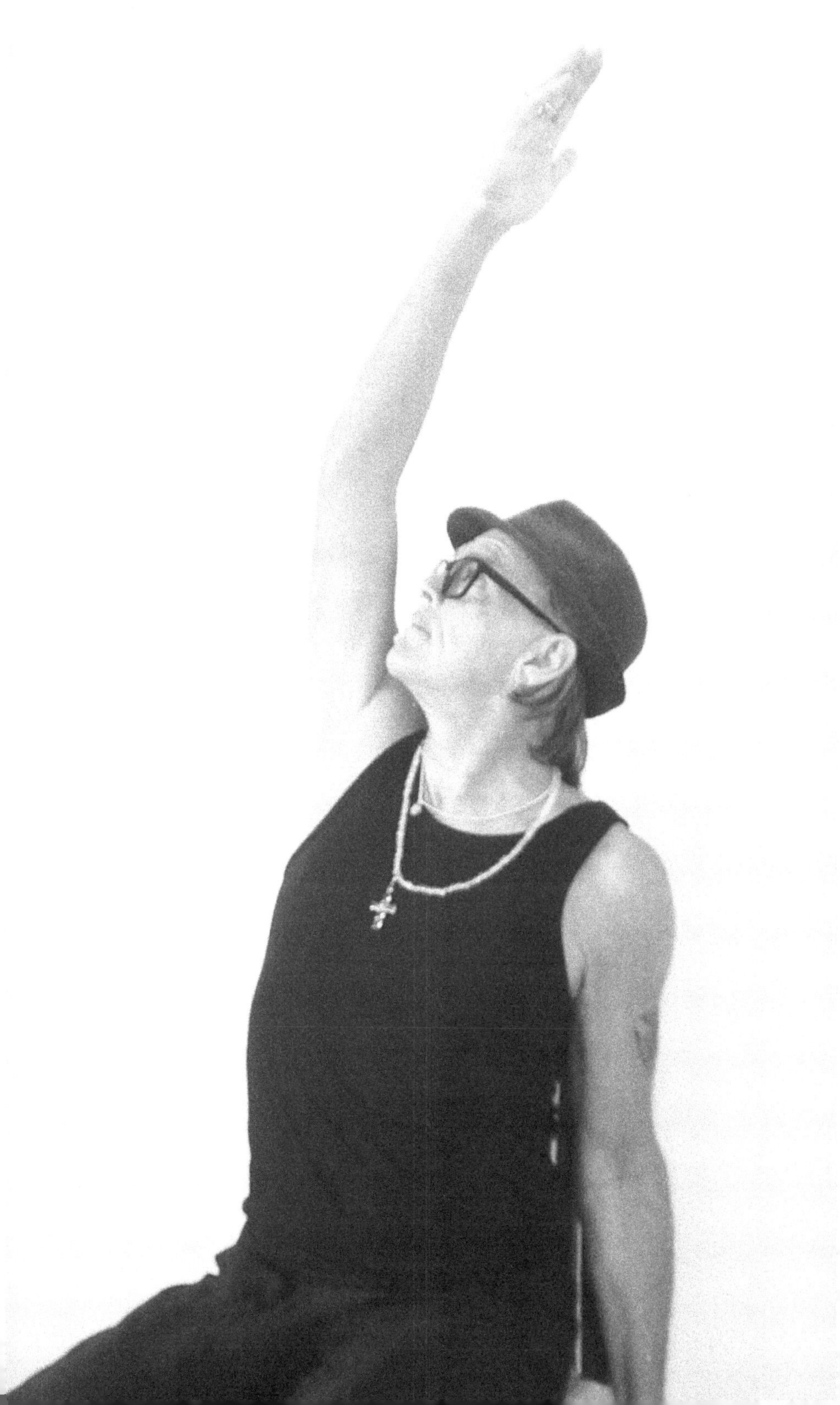

SPINAL TWIST

Twists help us restore and maintain the range of motion in our spine. Without focusing on the range of motion of our spine, we allow the muscles, tendons, ligaments, and fascia to shorten and stiffen, along with our joints gradually becoming harder.

Start in a seated mountain pose with your knees over your ankles, hip-width apart. Ensure your spine is straight. To begin the twist, take a deep breath in. Exhale as you twist your spine to the right. Place your left hand on the outside of your right knee and your right arm on the back of the chair. If possible, lengthen your spine with each inhale and, on the exhale, deepen the twist. Listen to your body so you only go as far as it can handle. Hold for 5 to 10 breaths before untwisting your spine. Repeat on the other side. Finish in mountain pose.

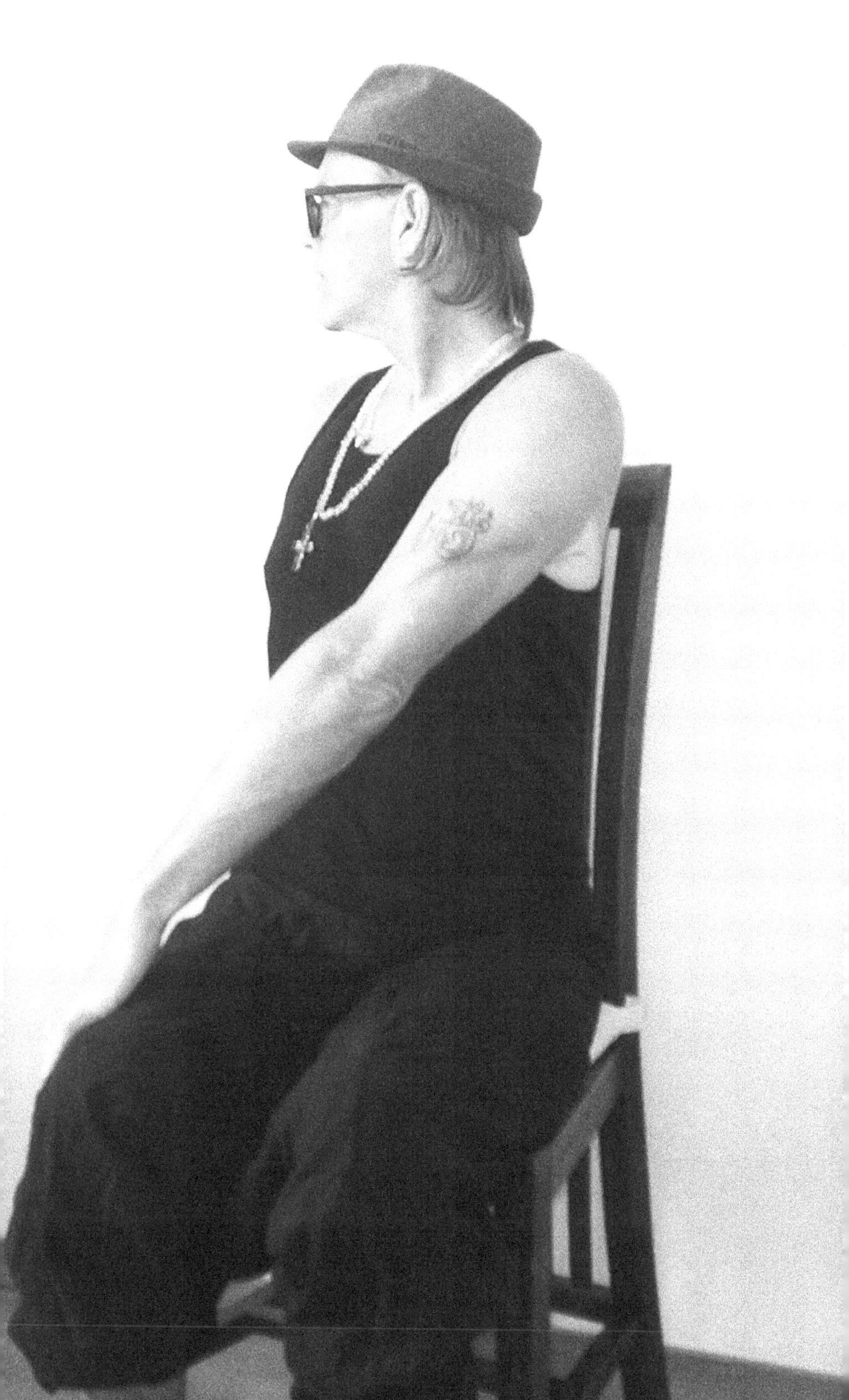

CHAIR YOGA WARM-UP FLOW

1. SUN SALUTATION

2. CAT

3. FORWARD BEND

4. SIDE BEND

5. SPINAL TWIST

Here's how you can combine the movements: Start your warm-up with the Sun Salutation, feeling the energy flow through your body. After completing the Sun Salutation, move on to practicing the Cat to warm up your spine. Once your spine is warmed up, proceed to a Forward Bend. The next step is to warm up your sides with the Side Bend. Finish with a Spinal Twist in both directions.

PIGEON

The Pigeon pose helps support flexibility and mobility in your hip flexors and lower back, two areas of your body that are often tight due to prolonged sitting. Stretching these muscles can help alleviate pain or tension in your lower back and hips.

Start by sitting on your chair with your buttocks near the edge of the seat. Place your right ankle on your left thigh or knee and rest your hands on your knee. Inhale and lengthen your spine. Hinge at your hips on the exhale to bring your chest toward your legs. Make sure not to round your back. Stay here for a few minutes before returning to the center.

TIPS

If you find it challenging to lift one leg to rest on the other, place a yoga block or a stack of yoga blocks on the inside of your supporting foot and place your bent leg on top of them.

PIGEON 2

Once you can manage the position with your hands resting on your knee, try the Pigeon pose with your hands in a prayer position as you lean forward.

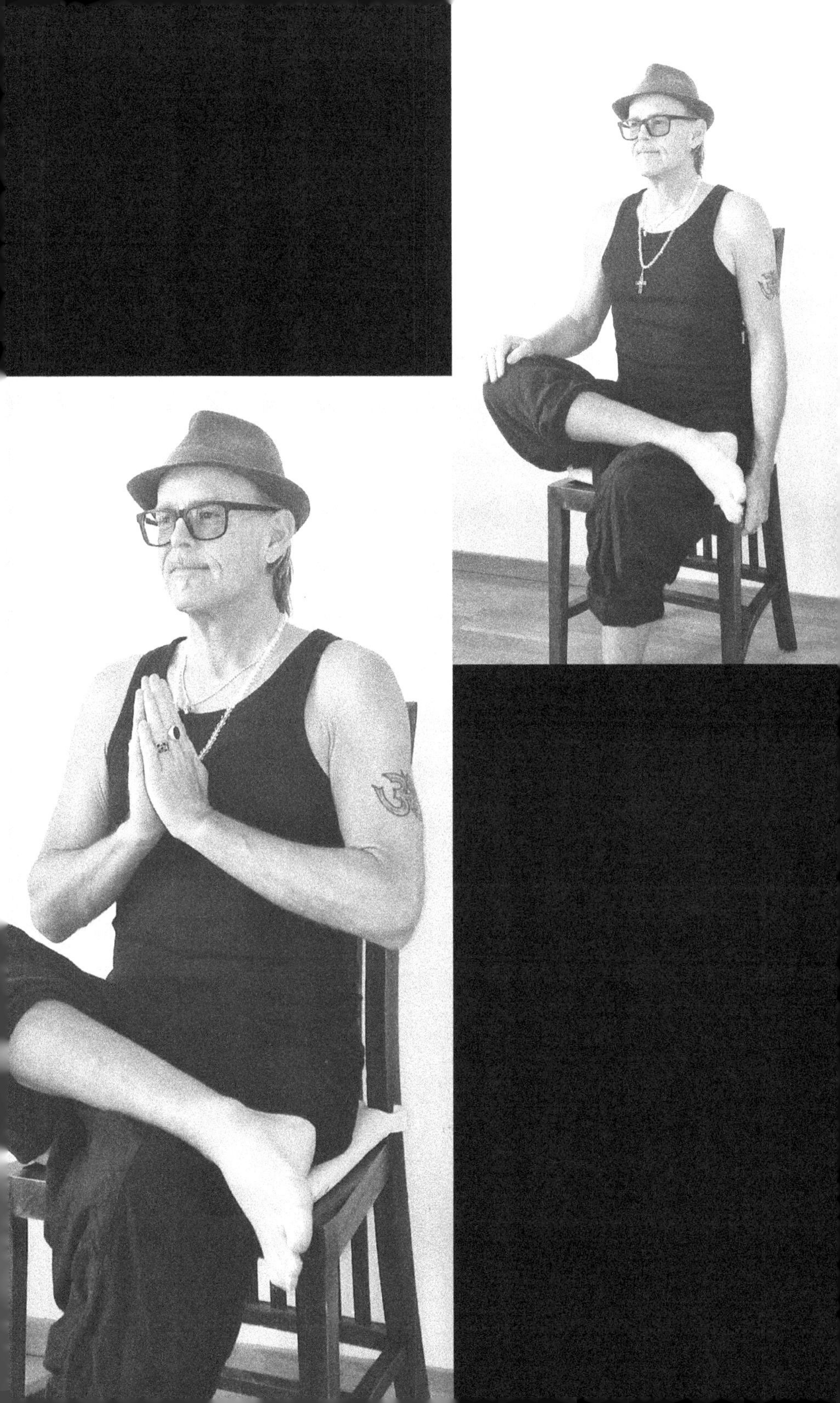

SINGLE-LEG FORWARD STRETCH

The seated single-leg forward stretch helps to stretch your calf muscles and hamstrings.

Sit on your chair with your buttocks as close to the front edge as possible. Extend your right leg in front of you with your toes pointing towards the ceiling. Inhale and bend forward to feel the stretch in your right leg. You can keep your hand resting on your shin or hold your toes if you can. Hold for a few breaths. Bring your right leg back and switch sides.

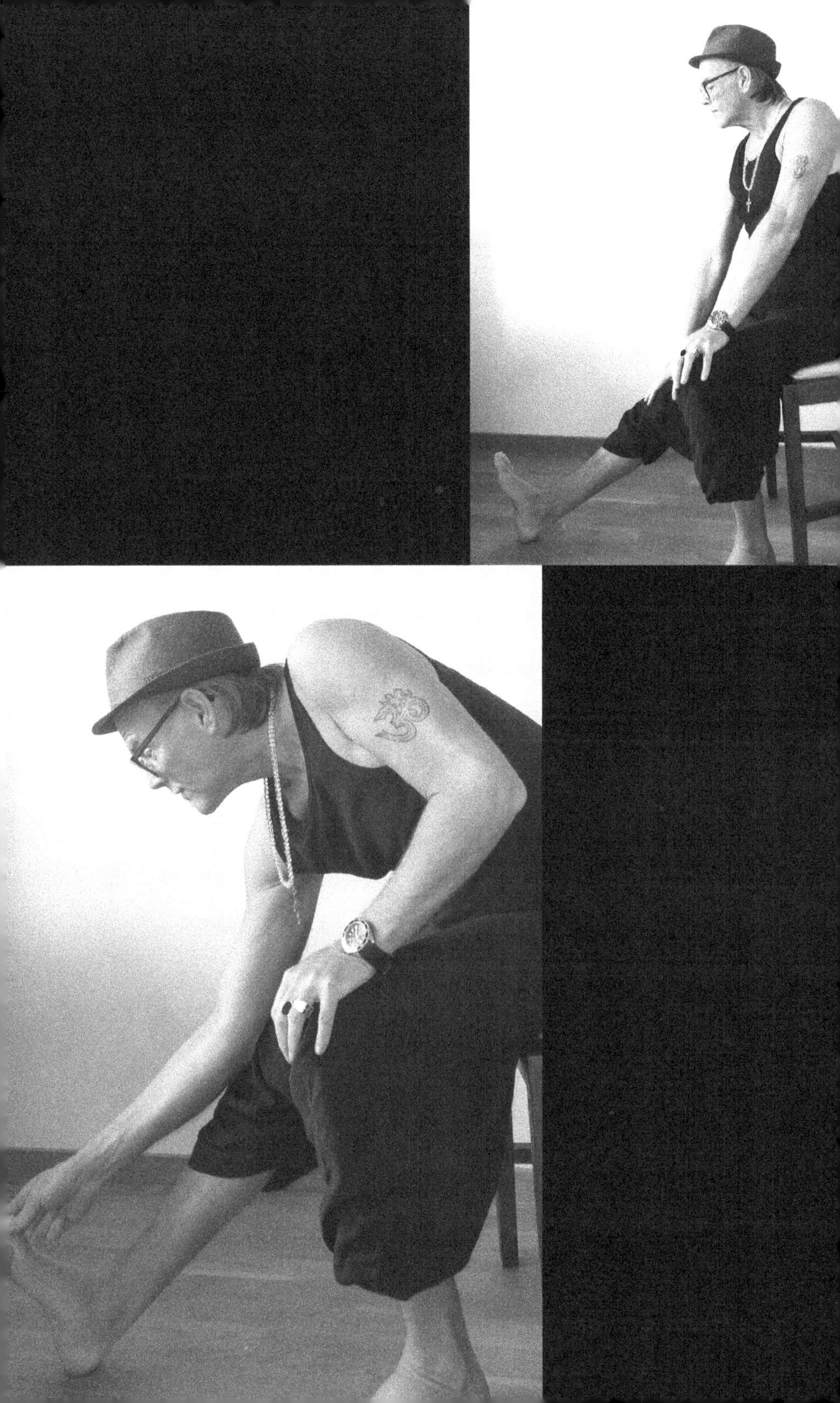

CHILD'S POSE

If yoga becomes too challenging, the child's pose is an excellent resting position. However, it's more than just a resting position. It can help relieve tension in your lower back and improve blood circulation. It can aid digestion and open up your hips, stretch your shoulders, energize the body, and calm the mind. You can use two chairs, a blanket, or a towel for this position.

Start in mountain pose. Exhale and lean forward, letting your fingertips touch the floor. Breathe deeply. Please stay in the position for as long as it feels comfortable. When you're ready, inhale and slowly roll up. Finish in mountain pose.

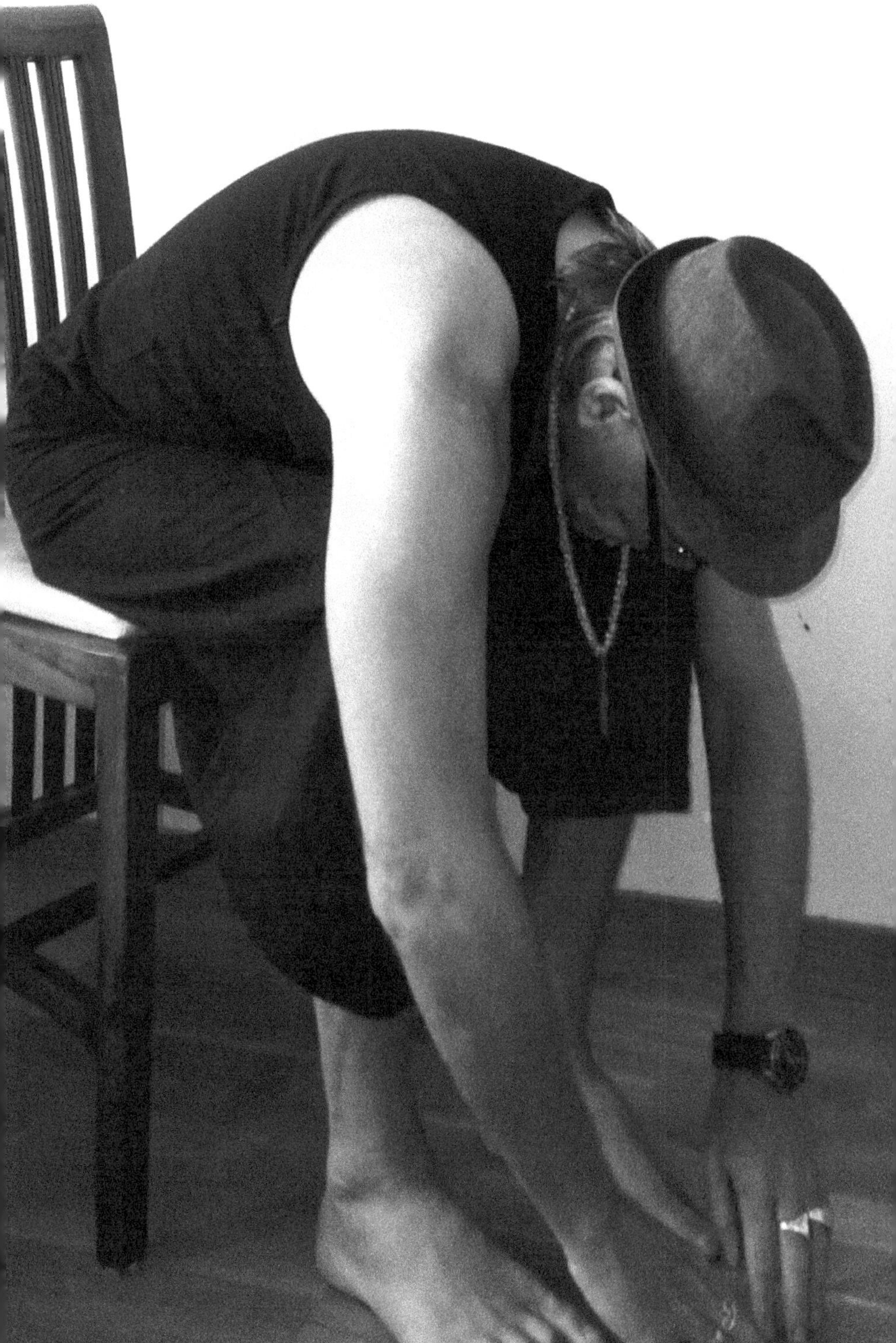

CHILD'S POSE WITH TWO CHAIRS

You can also choose to use two chairs for this position.

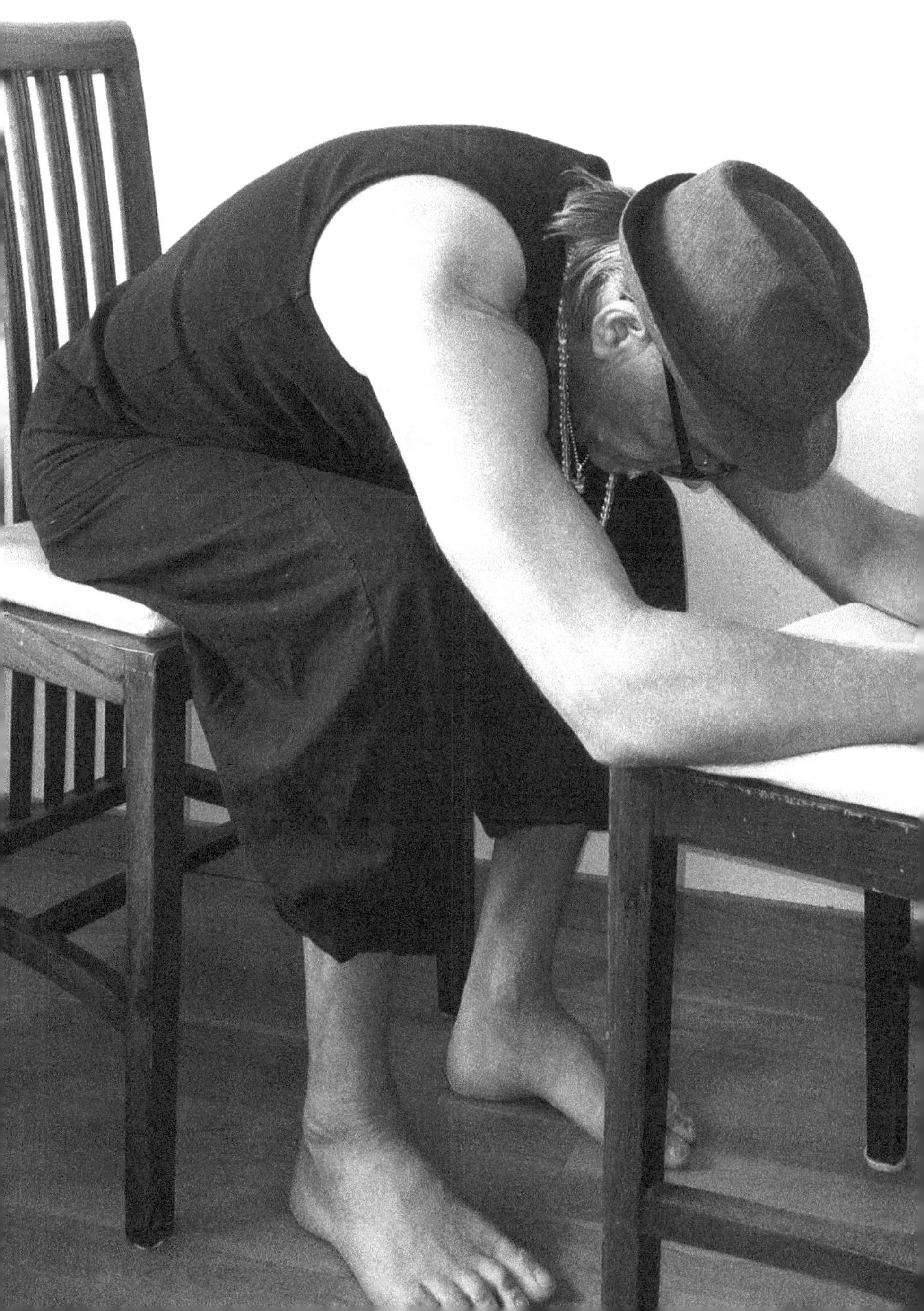

ENDING

You can conclude with the seated mountain pose at the end of your warm-up or chair yoga session. Sit on your chair and let your hands rest on your knees. Close your eyes. Take deep breaths and release all tension from your body. Listen to your breath and gaze toward the eyebrow center, visualizing a bright white light.

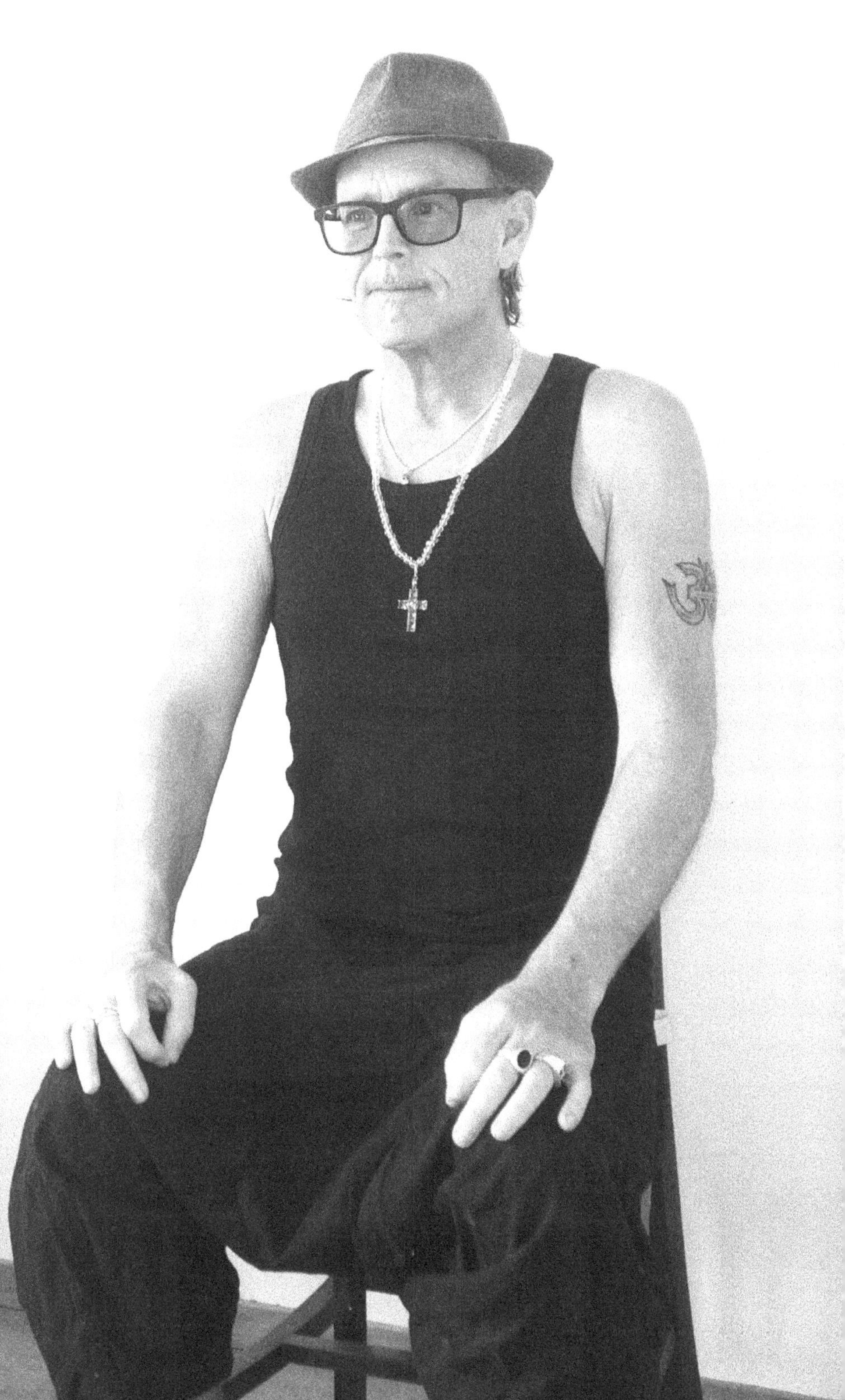

3

CHAIR YOGA FOR BETTER BALANCE

Improved balance is one of the many health benefits of practicing yoga. One can achieve increased stability, control, and body awareness by integrating various yoga poses and techniques.

Yoga Poses, particularly those requiring standing on one leg or performing balanced movements, engage and strengthen the muscles in the feet, ankles, legs, and core (Kannusamy et al., 2016). A study published in the Journal of Bodywork and Movement Therapies found that a 12-week yoga intervention improved balance in older adults by increasing muscle strength and stability (Roland et al., 2011).

Proprioception Training: Yoga promotes proprioception, the ability to understand the body's position in space. By performing various yoga poses that require fine-tuned movements and control over body position, practitioners develop a deeper awareness of their body and its movements (Shumway-Cook & Woollacott, 2007). It enhances the sense of balance and stability by improving the ability to respond to surface or body position changes.

Breathing and Relaxation: Yoga also focuses on breathing techniques and relaxation exercises that can reduce stress and tension in the body. By reducing stress levels and promoting relaxation, yoga can help relieve muscle tension and promote a more relaxed posture and balance (Cramer et al., 2013). A study published in the Journal of Geriatric Physical Therapy found that older adults participating in a six-week yoga intervention reported improved balance and reduced fall risk (Schmid et al., 2016).

Mental Focus and Presence: Yoga promotes mental presence and focus, crucial for maintaining balance and stability during movement. By cultivating mindful presence and concentration, practitioners can increase their ability to respond to external stimuli and maintain balance in various situations (Wayne & Fuerst, 2013).

In conclusion, yoga offers a comprehensive approach to improving balance by combining strength training, proprioception training, breathing exercises, and mental focus. Research shows that regular yoga practice can increase balance and stability and reduce fall risk in people of all ages.

REFERENCES

Cramer, H., Lauche, R., Haller, H., & Dobos, G. (2013). A systematic review and meta-analysis of yoga for low back pain. The Clinical Journal of Pain, 29(5), 450-460.

Kannusamy, P., Venugopal, V., & Sivaramakrishnan, H. (2016). Comparative effect of hatha yoga and physical exercise on static and dynamic balance in Thai community-dwelling older adults. Journal of Physical Therapy Science, 28(2), 635-640.

Roland, K. P., Jakobi, J. M., & Jones, G. R. (2011). Does yoga engender fitness in older adults? A critical review. Journal of Aging and Physical Activity, 19(1), 62-79.

Schmid, A. A., Van Puymbroeck, M., Koceja, D. M., DeBaun-Sprague, E., & Portz, J. D. (2016). Effect of a 12-week yoga intervention on fear of falling and balance in older adults: a pilot study. Archives of Physical Medicine and Rehabilitation, 97(10), 1520-1522.

Shumway-Cook, A., & Woollacott, M. (2007). Motor control: translating research into clinical practice. Lippincott Williams & Wilkins.

Wayne, P. M., & Fuerst, M. L. (2013). The Harvard Medical School guide to yoga: 8 weeks to strength, awareness, and flexibility. Da Capo Lifelong Books.

INSTRUCTIONS BEFORE THE YOGA SESSION

Cleanse the nose with a neti pot (a nasal rinsing can with lukewarm water and salt) or nasal spray. Do not eat heavy food approximately 2-3 hours before. Preferably, be vegetarian. Do not drink caffeine. All of this calms the mind and gets the blood and prana moving in the body. Sit relaxed with a straight back.

THE TREE

Stand with the right side facing the back of the chair, with your right hand resting on your back. Rotate your left leg out, lift your heel so the toes rest on the floor, and your heel rests against the inside of your right leg. When ready, raise your left foot to rest fully against your right leg above your ankle or calf muscle. Lift your left arm over your head and hold. Lower and switch sides. Once you master the position, try challenging yourself to let go of the chair and balance. You can also bring your foot to your thigh, making balancing a bit harder and deepening the stretch in your hip flexors.

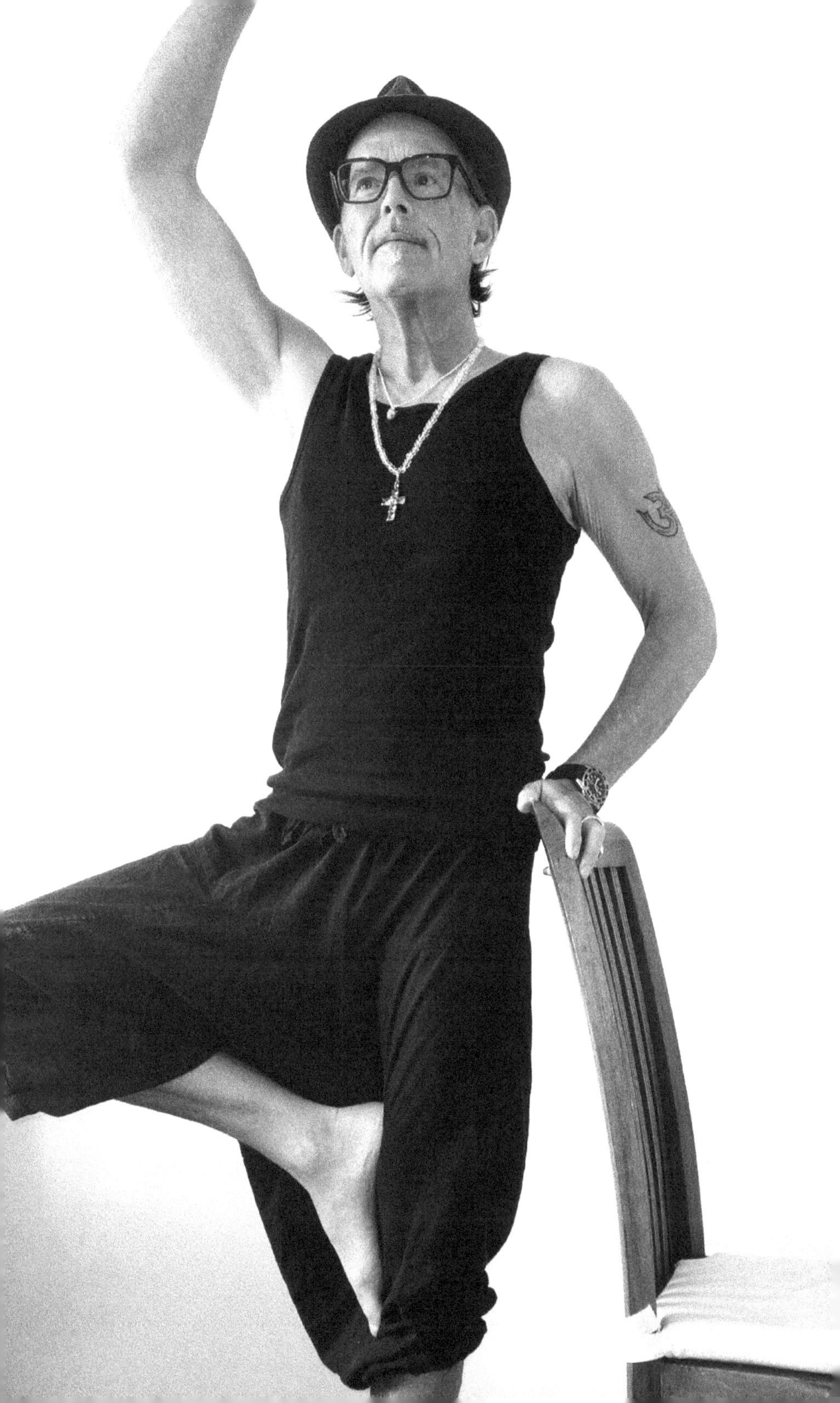

FOOT ON CHAIR

*Position the chair facing towards you and stand approxima-
tely two to three steps away from it. Place your left hand on
the chair's backrest as you place your right foot on the chair's
seat. Keep your right hand on your hip or lift your arm overhead. Hold for a few moments, then switch sides. Once you
master this position, you can challenge yourself by releasing
your grip on the chair and balancing without support.*

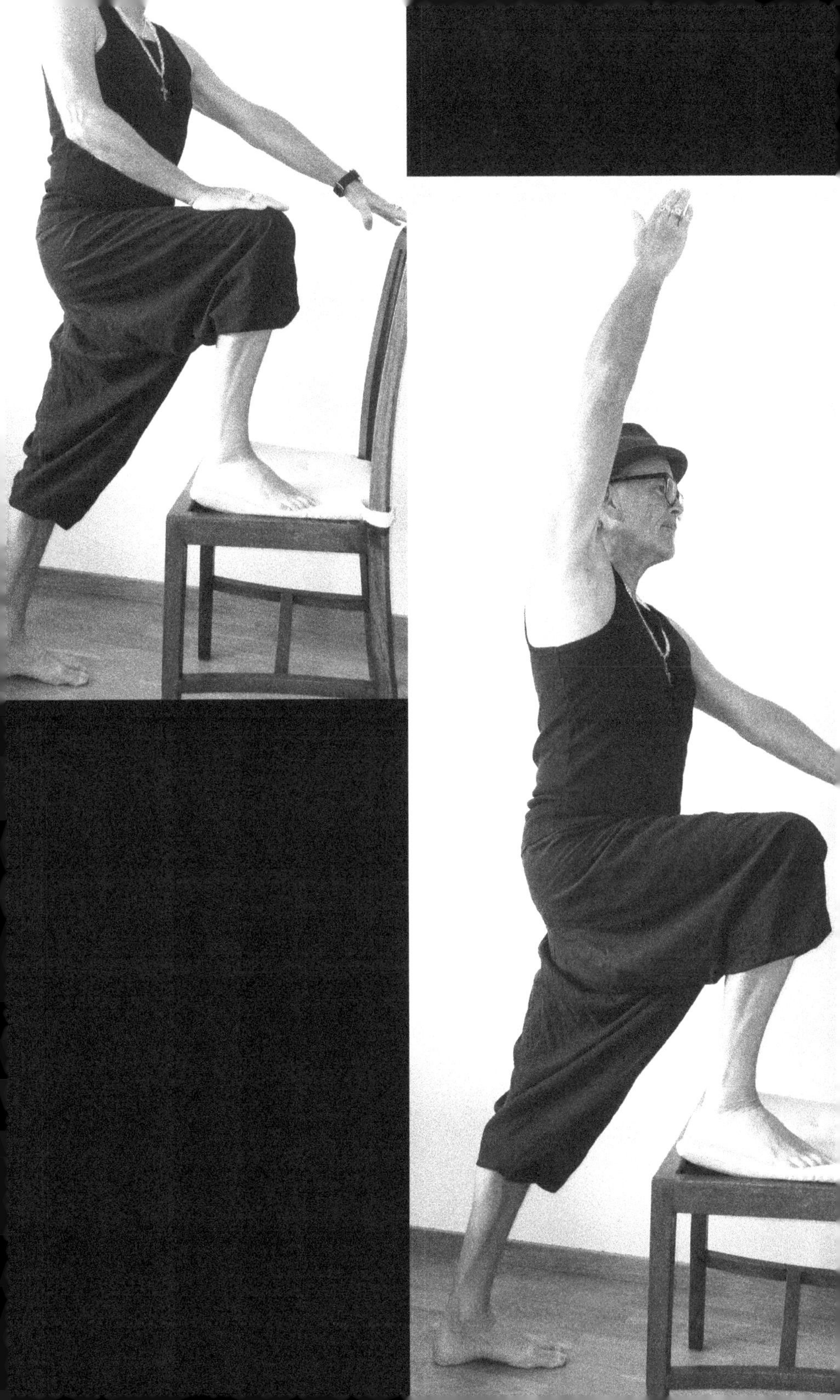

TRIANGLE

The triangle pose is a common foundational asana (yoga position). Since it challenges your balance and stability, you'll notice it stretching your hamstrings.

Position your chair facing towards you. Stand approximately three to four feet away from it on the left side with your feet hip-width apart. Rotate your left foot about 45 degrees while keeping your right foot facing the chair. Inhale as you lift your left arm to shoulder height. Extend your right arm towards the seat or backrest of the chair on the exhale. Hold for a few moments, then repeat on the other side. To further challenge yourself, you can gaze up towards the ceiling.

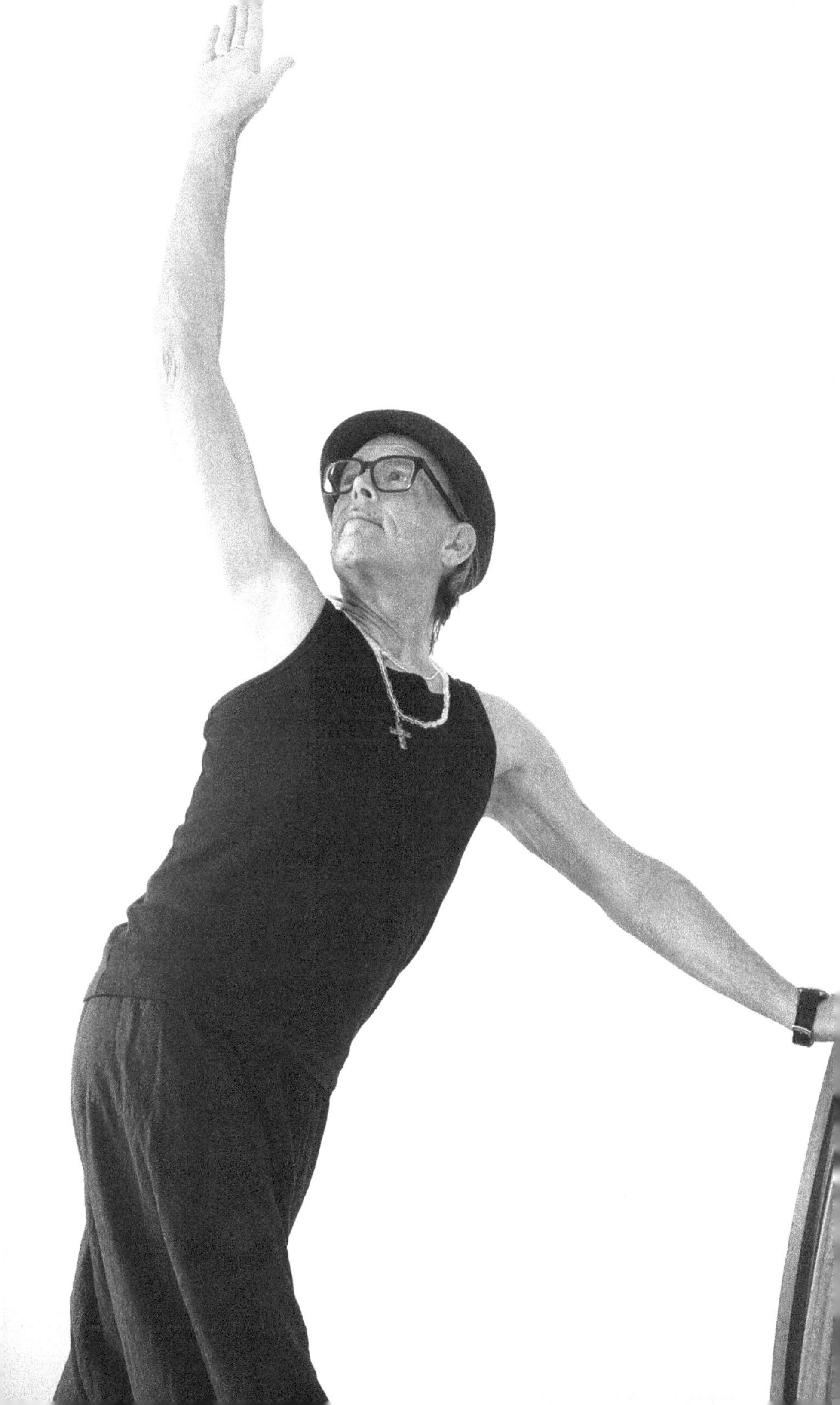

PALM TREE

This position is excellent for challenging your balance as you stand on your toes and stretch your arms, chest, core muscles, spine, and legs.

Stand behind your chair with your hands resting on the back. Rise onto your toes. Extend your left arm over your head as you shift your weight onto the right leg. You should notice the movement resembling a side stretch. Return to the center, place your raised arm back on the chair, then switch sides. Sway from side to side for a few breaths.

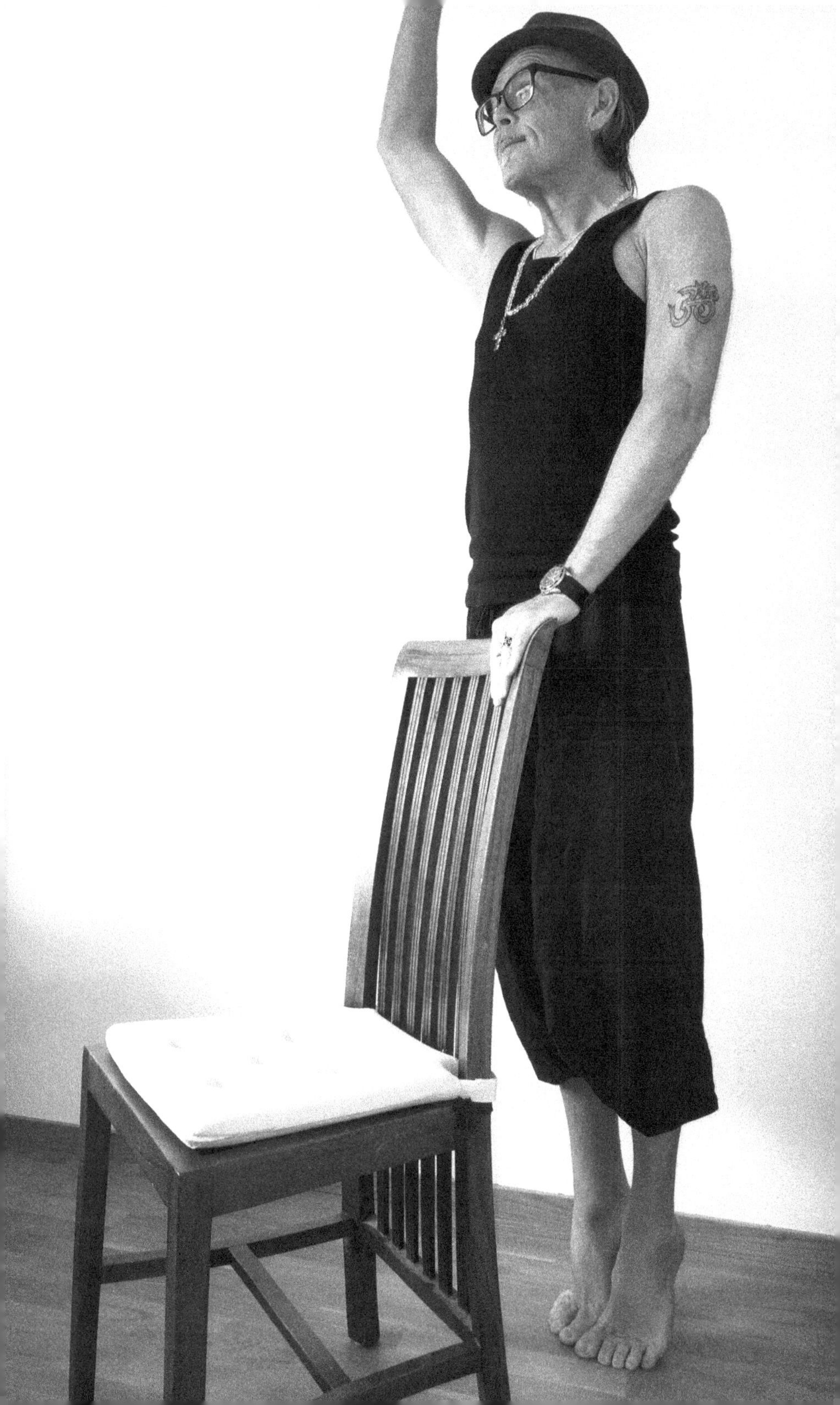

BALANCE CHAIR YOGA FLOW 1

Here's how to put together the first flow: stand next to your chair with your right hand holding the backrest for the tree pose.

Rotate your right foot into the ground and bend your left knee, placing the sole of your left foot on the inside of your right thigh. You can choose whether it feels better on your ankle, calf, or above the knee, but make sure it's not direct-ly on the knee. Lift your left arm overhead when your foot is comfortable, and balance here for a few breaths. Gently lower your left foot to the ground while holding onto the chair for support. Then, let your left-hand rest on the backrest for the foot-on-chair position.

Stand about two to three steps from the chair and place your right foot on the chair seat. For an extra challenge, place your right hand on your hip or lift your arm overhead. Balance here for a few breaths before transitioning to the triangle pose.

Place your right foot back on the ground while holding onto the chair with your left hand. Turn to face the front of your chair, place your feet shoulder-width apart, with your left foot facing the chair and your right foot pointing forward. Shift your right hip back, slide your left hand along the chair, and stretch your right arm toward the ceiling. It should create a nice straight line from your left hand to your right. Remem-

*ber to keep both legs straight and chest open. Hold this posi-
tion for a few breaths and then rise.*

*Return to face the back of your chair with your feet together,
resting your hands on the backrest for the palm tree pose.*

*As you inhale, rise onto your toes. As you exhale, shift your
weight onto the right leg and stretch your left arm overhead.
Lift your left heel off the ground to feel a nice side stretch. Inhale to return to the center, place your raised arm back on the
chair, and switch sides. Continue swaying from side to side for
a few breaths.*

THE ANGLE

The angle pose is an essential seated position similar to the sitting mountain pose, except your legs are extended in front of you. This pose helps stretch your calves and hamstrings while increasing spine awareness.

Sit close to the edge of your chair with your legs extended in front of you and your toes pointing toward the ceiling. Place your hands behind the edge of the chair with your fingers facing forward. Press into your hands to gently push your upper body forward until you feel a stretch in your calves and hamstrings. Hold for a few moments, and then release.

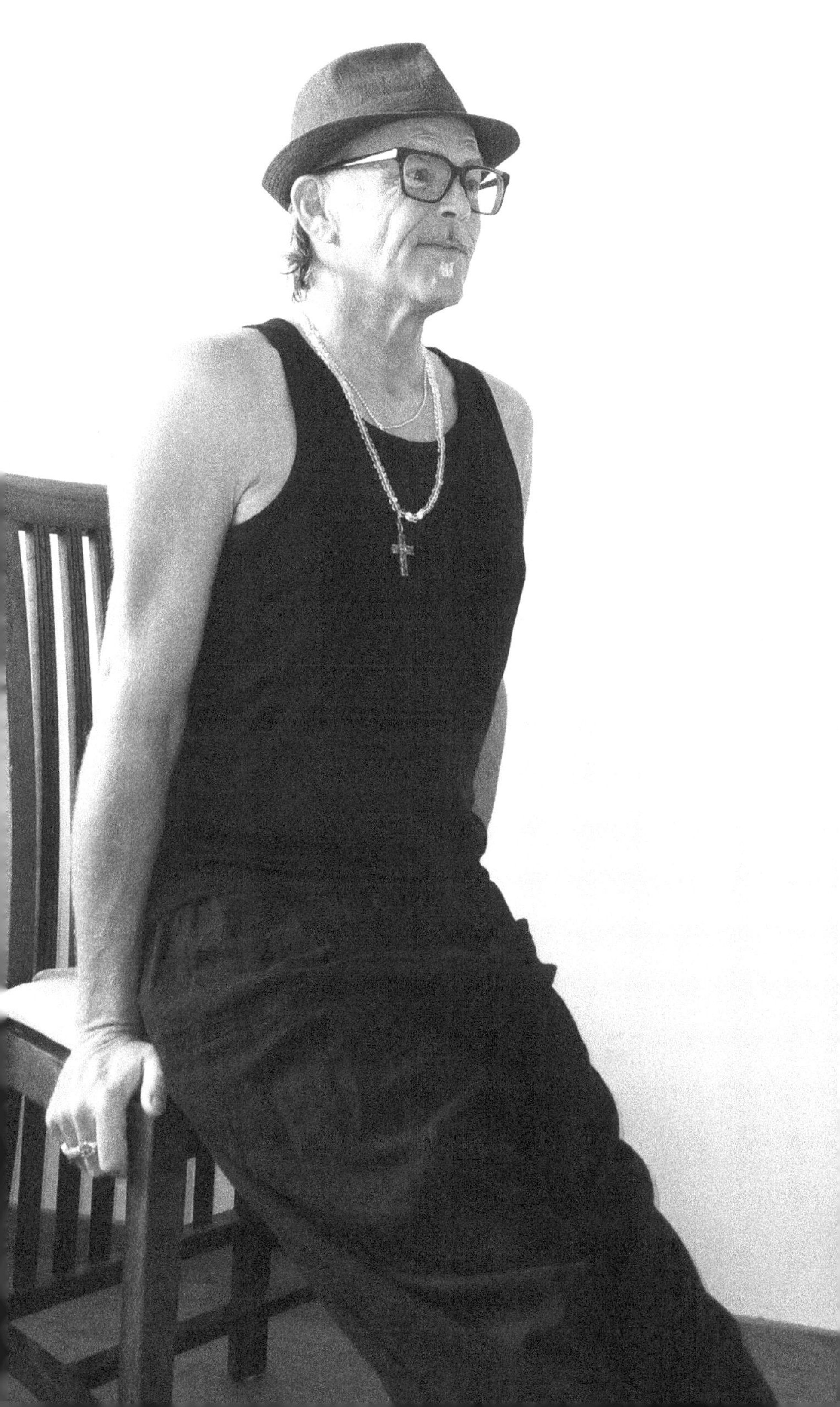

BOUND ANGLE

The bound angle pose is a variation of the butterfly pose and is excellent for strengthening and improving flexibility in your thighs, knees, and groin. It's also a position that can help alleviate sciatica and lower back pain symptoms. You can use a pair of yoga blocks or a rolled-up cushion to support your ankles for this yoga position.

Sit close to the edge of your chair with your yoga blocks or a rolled-up cushion stacked in front of you. Your hands can rest on the seat or your thighs. Rest the outsides of your ankles on the block and let your knees fall to the sides. Hold the position for a minute. You can also use a second chair instead of the yoga blocks.

Sit close to the edge of your chair with the other chair in front of you. Your hands can rest on the seat or your thighs, or you can place them in a prayer position. Rest the outsides of your ankles on the edge of the other chair and let your knees fall to the sides.

This sequence also includes forward bending and seated pigeon pose.

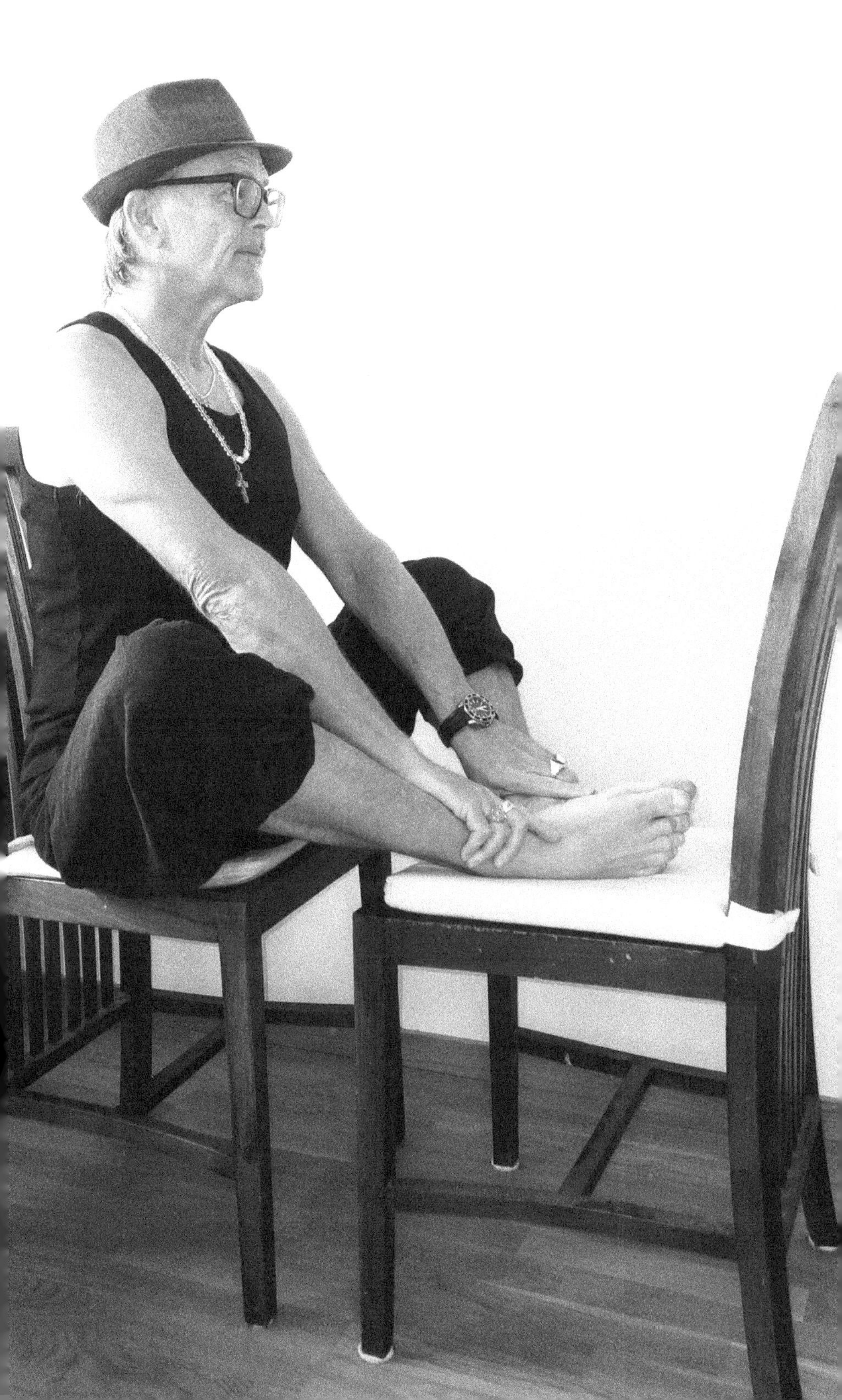

BOUND ANGLE IN PRAYER POSITION

Bound angle pose with hands in prayer position.

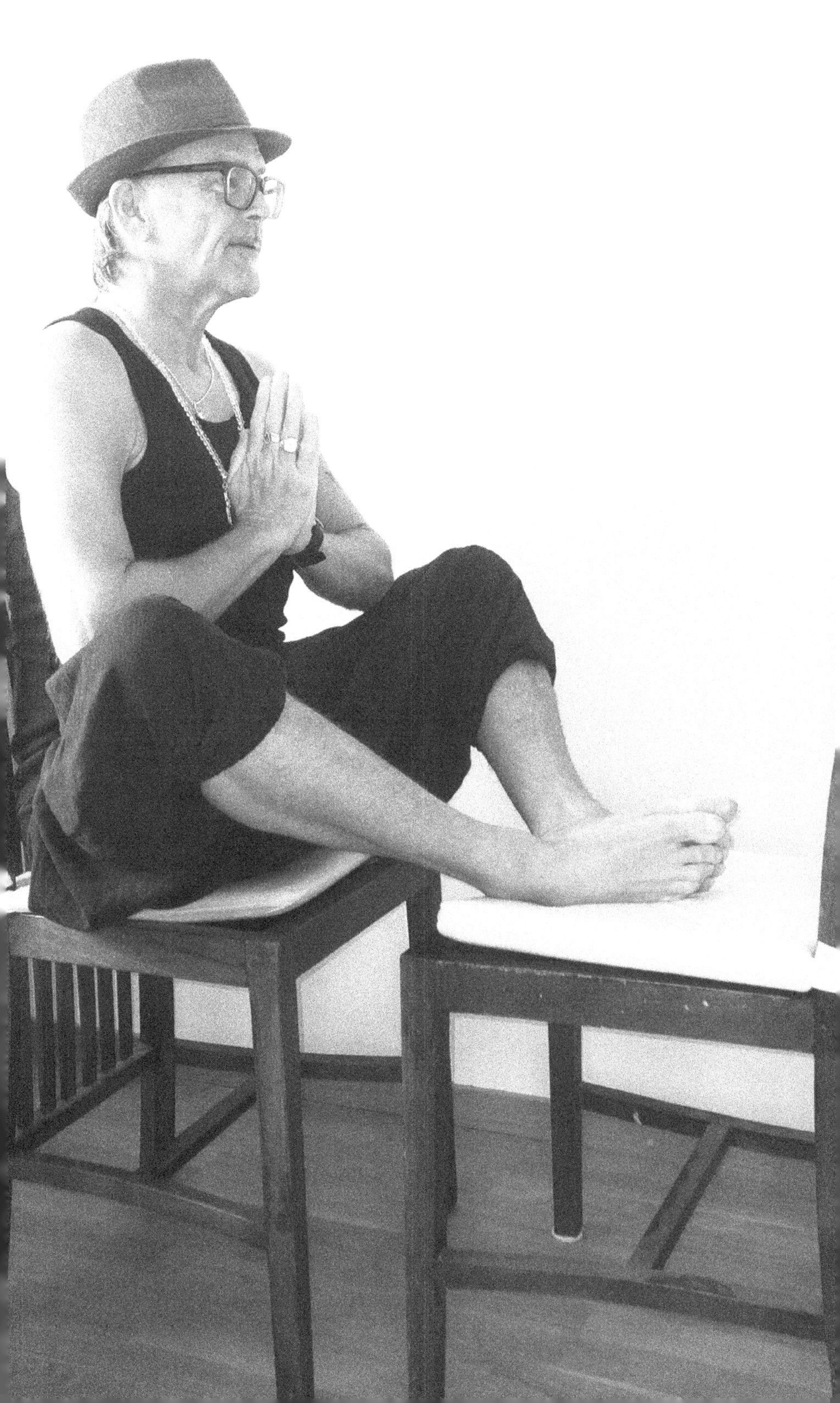

FLOW FOR BALANCE CHAIR YOGA 2

First, sit comfortably on your chair with your feet firmly on the ground, about hip-width apart, for a forward fold.

Reach your arms up toward the ceiling on a deep inhale, elongating your spine. As you exhale, bend forward from your hips, letting your hands rest on your shins, ankles, or the floor, depending on your flexibility. Let your head hang down briefly before moving into the angle.

Slowly roll up your body, one vertebra at a time, until you're sitting tall again. Extend your legs straight before you when sitting upright, keeping your feet flexed and active. Place your hands behind your seat on the chair with fingers pointing forward and press into your hands to gently press your torso forward until you feel a stretch in your calves and hamstrings.

To move into the pigeon pose, bend your right knee and place your right foot flat on the ground. Then, place your left ankle over your right knee. You can stay in the position for a while if it feels good. If you want a deeper stretch, gently lean forward from your hips. You should feel this in your left hip for a good stretch and balance challenge.

After a few breaths in pigeon pose, gently uncross your leg, returning your foot to the ground. Scoot slightly forward on your chair to allow space for your feet to come together. Place the underside of your foot on your yoga block or chair and let your knees fall to the sides. Hold for a couple of breaths. Then, switch sides and repeat.

WARRIOR 1

Warrior 1 strengthens your legs by opening your chest and hips and stretching your arms and legs. This pose also helps improve your circulation and respiration. As you stand in warrior, feel the energy flowing through you as you ground yourself to the floor.

Begin by sitting on your chair in a mountain pose. Turn to your right to sit on the side of your chair. Keep your right foot facing forward, and extend your left leg to the side, aiming to keep your left foot on the ground with your hips turning to the right. Take a deep breath and lift both arms overhead with palms facing inward. On the exhale, shift your left leg behind you as far as is comfortable.

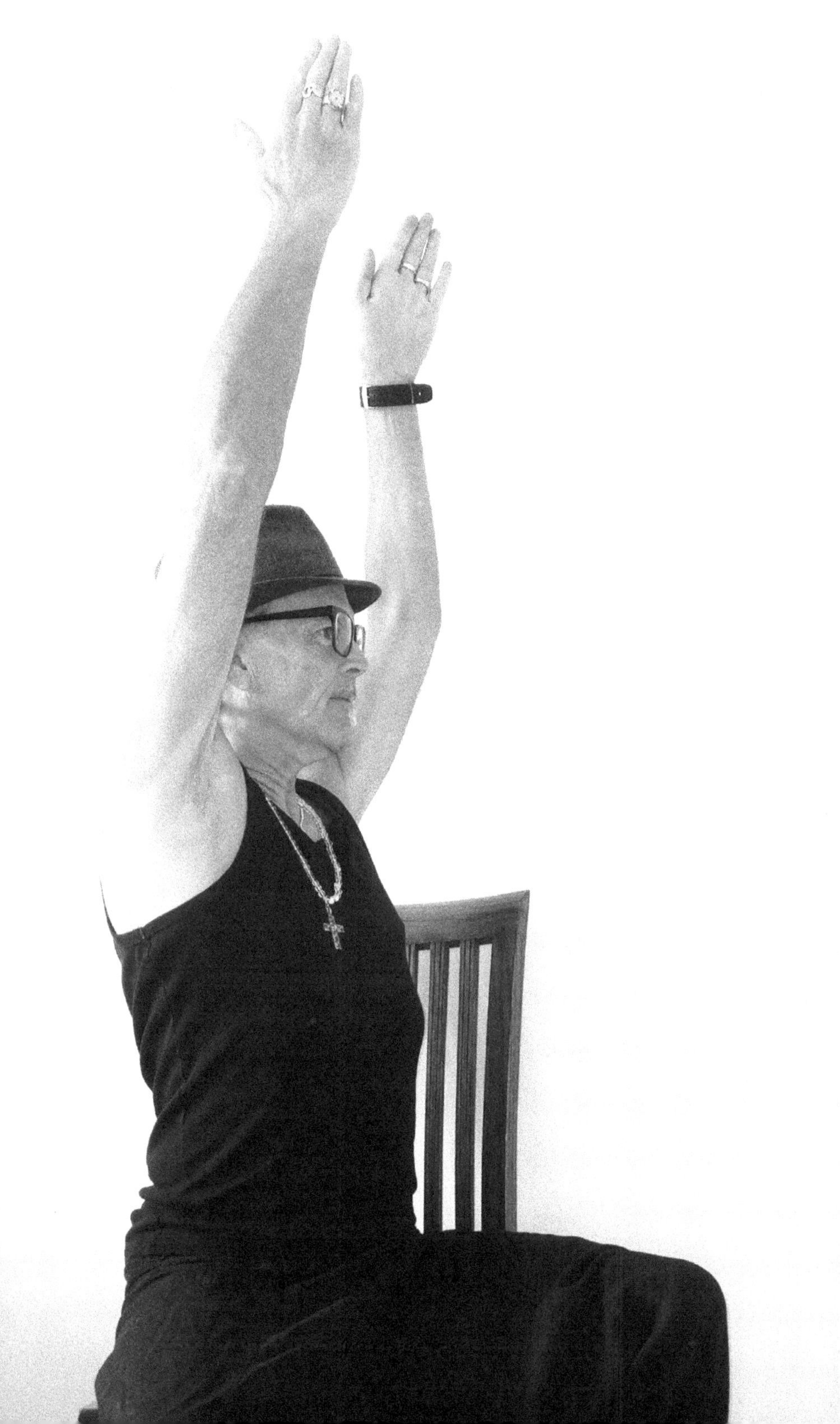

WARRIOR 2

Warrior 2 takes the essential warrior position to the next level, providing power, strength, and vision as you ground yourself to the earth. In addition to its symbolic nature, the position helps create flexibility in the hips and legs. You can transition into this position from Warrior 1.

From Warrior 1 on the right side, inhale as you rotate your torso toward the front of your chair. Exhale and bring your arms to shoulder height with palms facing the floor.

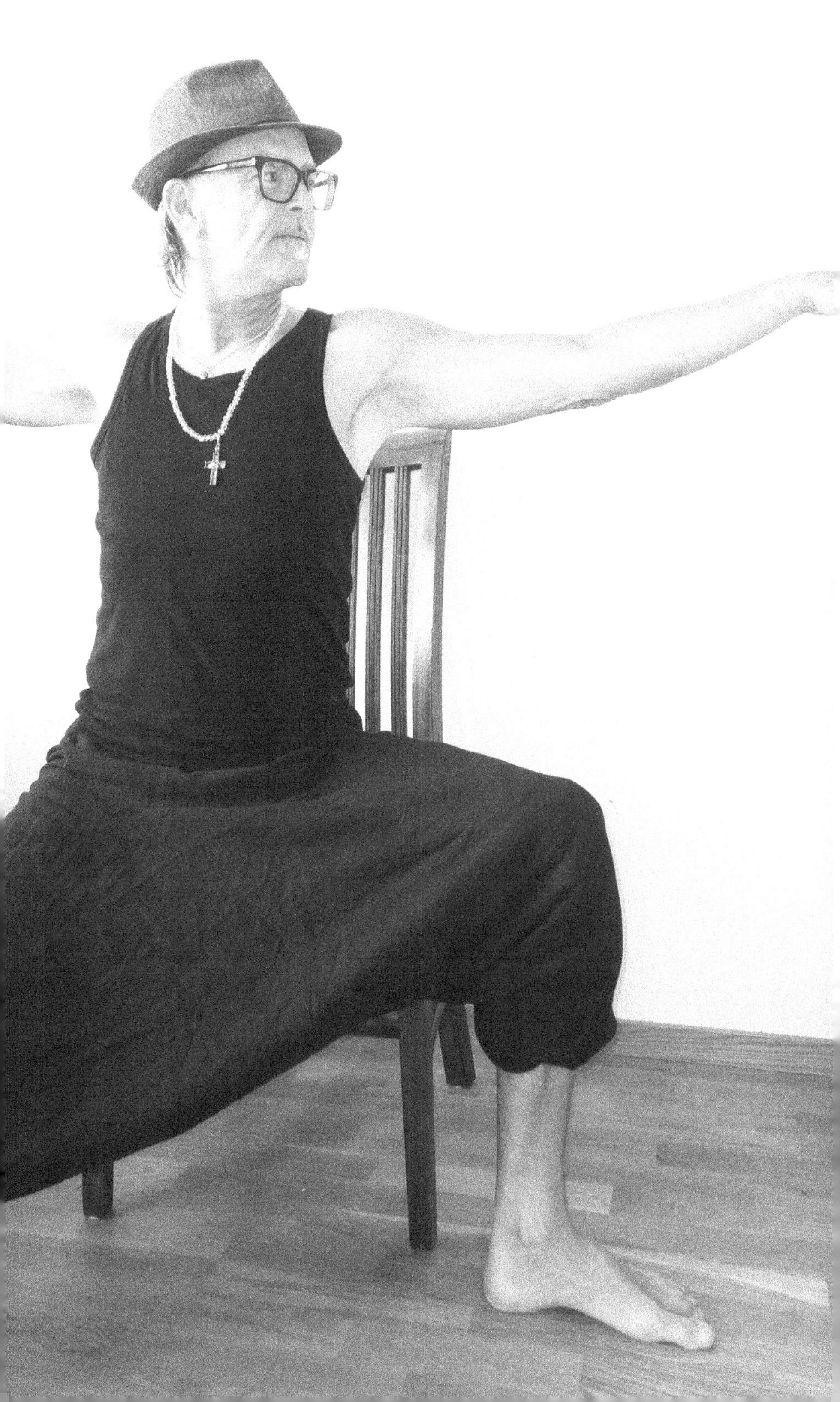

REVERSE WARRIOR

Reverse Warrior helps strengthen your legs as you open the side of your body from a side bend. It also improves the mobility of your spine, core, and balance strength. This position is also very energizing, supporting your respiration and circulation throughout your body. You can flow into this position from Warrior 2.

From Warrior 2, let your left arm come down behind you. Inhale and lift your right arm towards the ceiling as you lean to the side. Rest your left hand on your left leg for support. To return to the starting position, draw in your legs and turn to sit on the front edge of your chair to return to the seated mountain position.

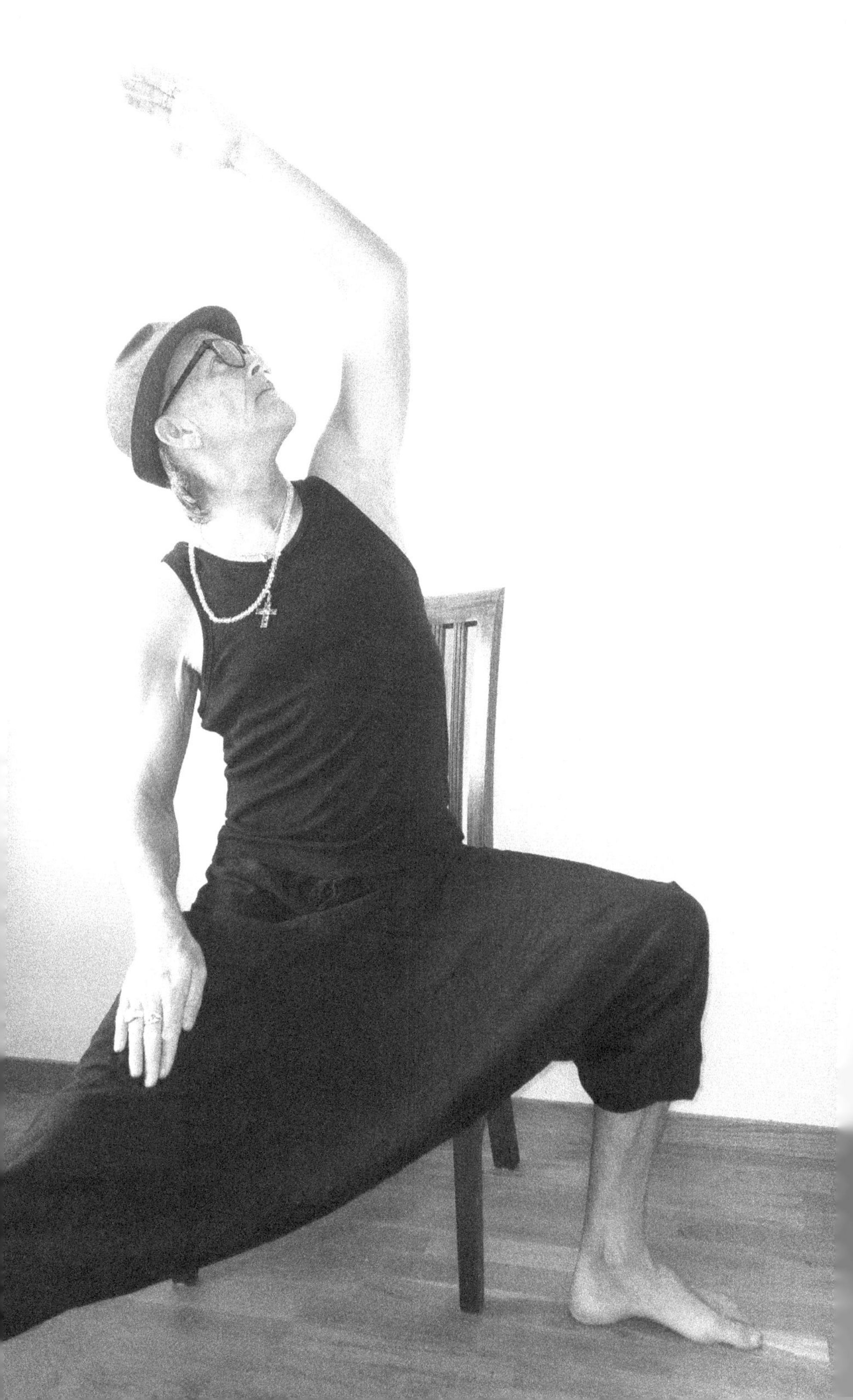

COBRA

Seated Cobra is an active position that energizes the upper body, strengthens and tones the wrists, arms, and abdominal muscles, and relieves pain and discomfort in the lower back.

Place your chair in front of you and against a wall to prevent it from moving. Alternatively, you can place your chair on a yoga mat. Lean forward and place your hands on your chair to hold onto the edges. Step back with your feet to come into the plank position. Inhale as you bend your arms, lower your shoulders, and arch your back to open up your chest to go into an exploratory position and look up. To release, exhale, and draw your hips back towards your heels to come into the child's pose.

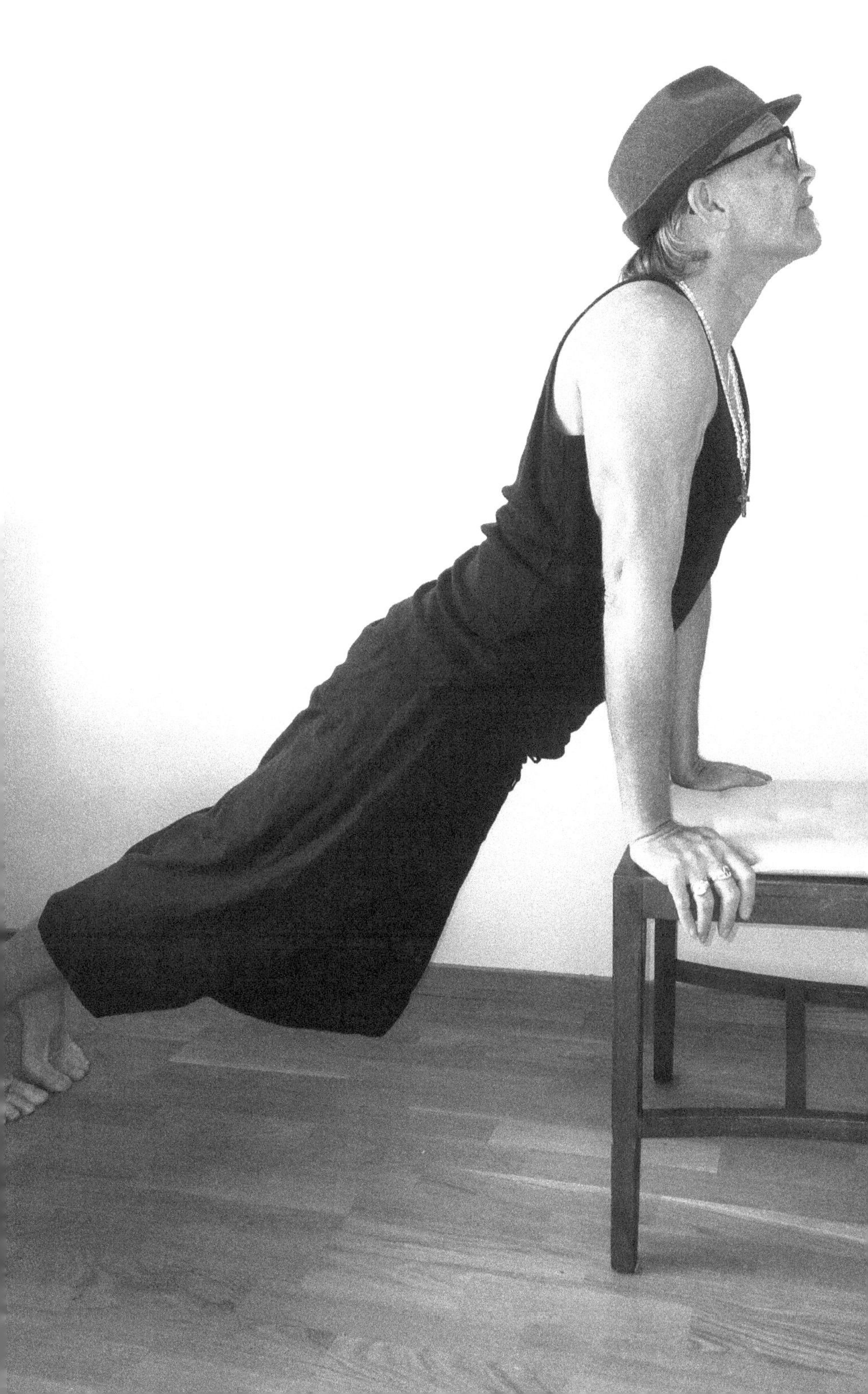

STANDING MOUNTAIN

Stand before or behind your chair and lean to rest your hands on the seat or backrest. Take a few steps back from the chair. Ensure your spine is straight, and your feet are hip-width apart. As you press your hands into the chair, roll your shoulders back and down away from your ears. Stay here and breathe deeply for three to five breaths. On your final inhale, step back towards your chair and slowly roll up to a standing position.

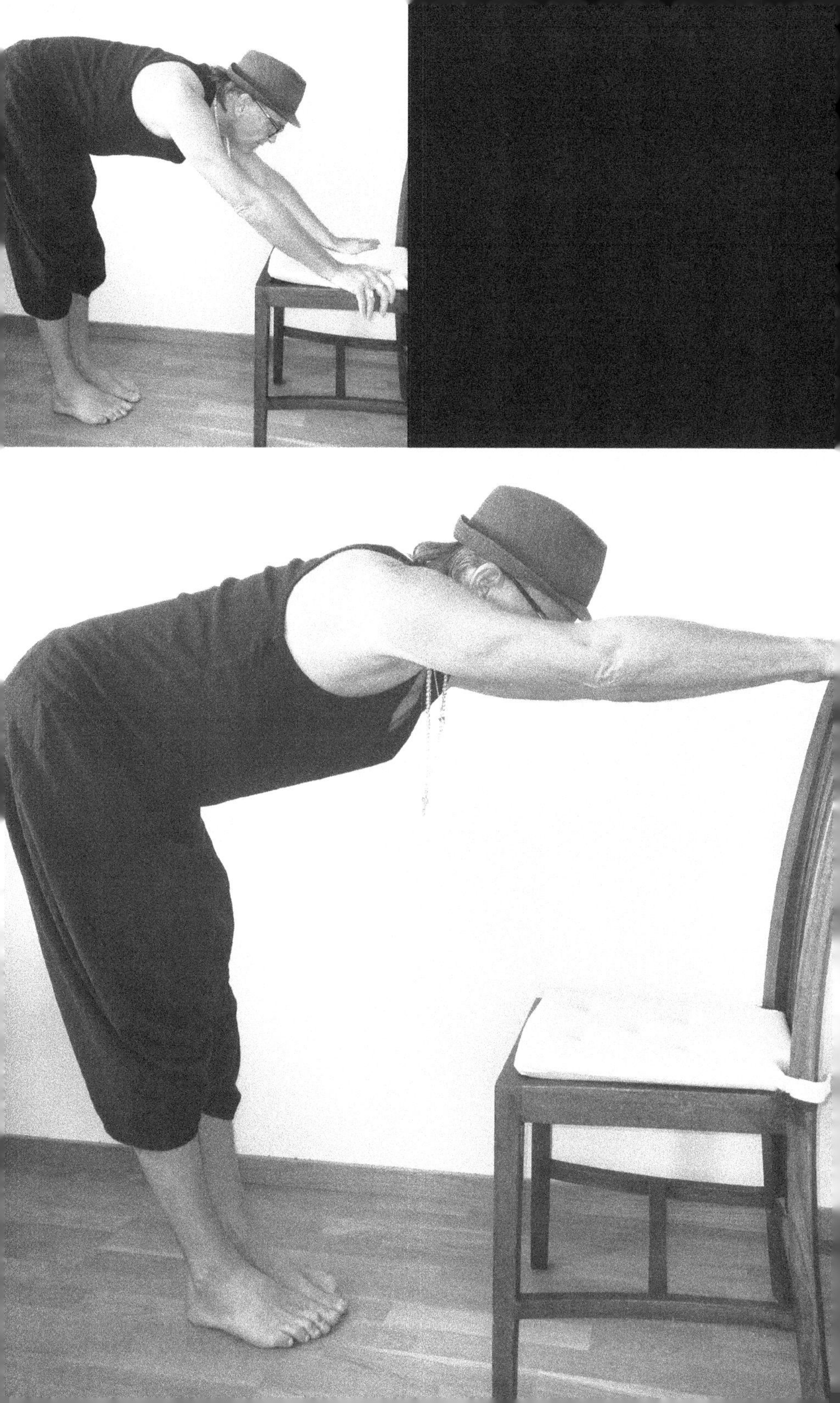

FLOW FOR BALANCE CHAIR YOGA 3

We begin with Warrior 1. Sit up tall on the edge of your chair. Rotate to the right so that your right leg is bent over the side of the chair and your right foot is flat on the floor. Extend your left leg behind you, toes pointing back and resting on the ground. Sweep your arms up towards the sky and take a moment to find your balance. While maintaining your leg positions, rotate your upper body to the left, lowering your arms to the sides at shoulder height, your right arm pointing forward, and your left arm pointing backward for Warrior 2.

Maintain your leg positions. Lower your left arm down to rest on the back of your left leg, and stretch your right arm up towards the sky for Reverse Warrior, creating a nice stretch on your right side. Remember to keep the right knee bent and maintain balance.

To transition into Standing Mountain, lower your right arm down and rotate your body back to the front of the chair to stand up. Place your chair in front of you (either on a yoga mat or against a wall to prevent it from moving) and take two to three steps back before bending forward at the hips to place your hands on the seat about shoulder-width apart to form an excellent "V" shape with your hips as the highest point. Press your palms into the chair, draw in your abdomen, and push your hips back. Your head should be in line with your arms. Hold for two more breaths. On your final exhale, simul-

taneously lower your hips and lift your chest until your body is about 45 degrees from the ground for Cobra.

Once you feel steady, inhale and lift your chest until you have a slight bend in your back. Exhale to deepen the backbend to your comfort level. On your final exhale, slowly reverse the position to pass through Standing Mountain before slowly rolling up to a standing position. Then, switch sides and repeat.

4

CHAIR YOGA FOR SOFTER JOINTS

Yoga is known for its many health benefits, one of which is the ability to soften joints and increase mobility. By practicing yoga regularly, participants can experience an improvement in joint flexibility and mobility, which can have positive effects on physical and mental health.

Stretching and muscle relaxation: One of the primary mechanisms through which yoga softens the joints is stretching muscles and connective tissue. Many yoga poses involve stretching and elongating muscles and tendons around the joints, promoting increased mobility and reducing tension and stiffness. A study published in the Journal of Physical Therapy Science found that regular yoga significantly improved participants' flexibility (Baptista et al., 2014).

Increased circulation: Yoga also promotes improved circulation throughout the body, which can help reduce inflammation and promote the healing process in the joints. When muscles are stretched and activated during yoga poses, blood flow to the area is stimulated, which can improve joint health and flexibility (Field, Diego, & Sanders, 2001).

Strengthening of muscles around the joints: In addition to stretching and relaxing the muscles, yoga also strengthens the muscles around the joints. By strengthening the muscles surrounding and supporting the joints, yoga can help increase stability and protect the joints from injuries and overexertion (Telles et al., 2016).

Breathing exercises and relaxation: Yoga often includes breathing exercises and relaxation techniques that can reduce stress and tension in the body. The joints can move freely without pain or discomfort when the body is relaxed and free from tension (Gard et al., 2014).

Improved proprioception: Yoga also promotes improved proprioception, which is understanding the body's position in space. By practicing various balanced and coordinated yoga poses, practitioners develop a deeper awareness of their joints and their movements, which can reduce the risk of injuries and increase flexibility (Wayne & Fuerst, 2013).

In summary, yoga offers a holistic approach to making the joints softer by combining stretching, muscle relaxation, increased circulation, muscle strength, and relaxation exercises. Research shows that regular yoga practice can result in improved joint health and increased mobility, which can help reduce the risk of joint-related problems and improve quality of life.

REFERENCES

Baptista, A. S., Silva, A. M., & Mazini Filho, M. L. (2014). Effect of 12 weeks of yoga training on the somatometric parameters and body composition of women. Journal of Physical Therapy Science, 26(12), 1921–1926.

Field, T., Diego, M., & Sanders, C. (2001). Exercise is positively related to adolescents' relationships and academics. Adolescence, 36(141), 105.

Gard, T., Noggle, J. J., Park, C. L., Vago, D. R., & Wilson, A. (2014). Potential self-regulatory mechanisms of yoga for psychological health. Frontiers in Human Neuroscience, 8, 770.

Telles, S., Sharma, S. K., Yadav, A., & Singh, N. (2016). Immediate effect of three yoga breathing techniques on performance on a letter-cancellation task. Perceptual and Motor Skills, 122(1), 187–195.

Wayne, P. M., & Fuerst, M. L. (2013). The Harvard Medical School guide to yoga: 8 weeks to strength, awareness, and flexibility. Da Capo Lifelong Books.

INSTRUCTIONS BEFORE THE YOGA SESSION

Cleanse the nose with a neti pot (a nasal rinsing can with lukewarm water and salt) or nasal spray. Refrain from eating heavy food approximately 2-3 hours before. Preferably, be vegetarian. Do not drink caffeine. All of this calms the mind and gets the blood and prana moving in the body. Sit relaxed with a straight back.

INVERTED CHAIR

Sit in the mountain pose, with your buttocks as close to the edge as possible. Rest your hands on your thighs. Inhale and lift your arms over your head with the palms facing each other and fingers pointing towards the ceiling. Exhale and press your weight through your heels to partially rise from your chair. Your end position should be a high squat where your legs are at about a 45-degree angle. Ensure that your spine remains straight with your neck in line with it. Hold three to five breaths and then slowly sit back on the chair, returning to the mountain pose.

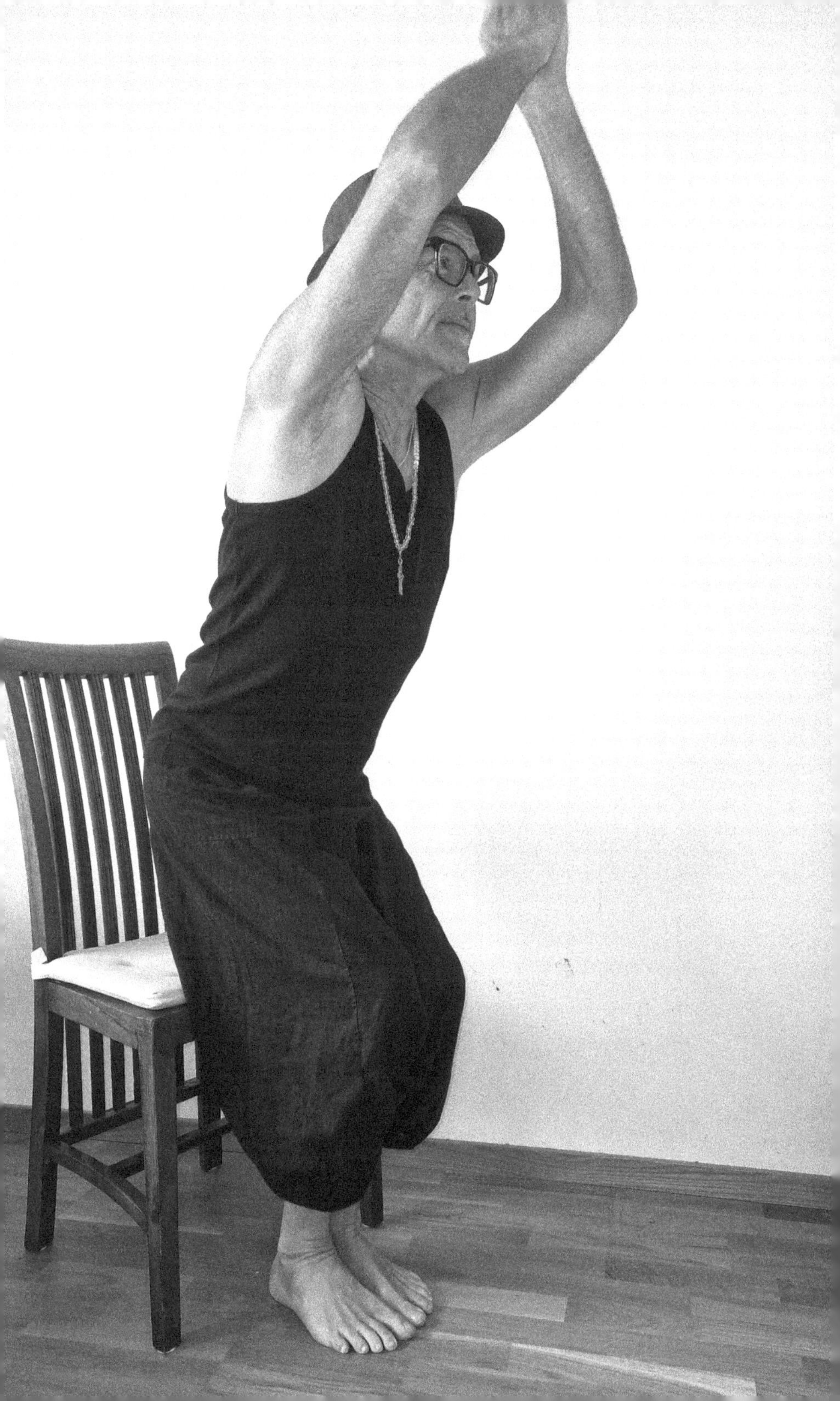

FLOW FOR SOFTER JOINTS 1

Start by sitting upright at the edge of your chair with your feet on the floor and your hands on your thighs. As you inhale, arch your back and press your chest forward for the cat pose. As you exhale, round your back, draw in your belly, and let your head sink forward. Continue to flow between these two movements synchronized with your breath. From the cat's position, gently come back to a neutral seated position.

Sit upright for spinal twisting, and as you exhale, twist your upper body to the right, placing your right hand on the back of the chair and your left hand on your right knee. Look over your right shoulder, hold for a few breaths, then inhale to return to the center. From the center, rotate to the right so that your right leg is bent over the side of the chair and your right foot is flat on the floor for Warrior 2.

Extend your left leg behind you, toes pointing backward and resting on the floor. Extend your arms to the sides at shoulder height, with your right arm pointing forward and your left arm pointing backward, and gaze over your right fingers. Hold for a few breaths. Then, rotate back with both feet back on the ground.

To enter the Reverse Chair, scoot a little towards the edge of your chair, keep your feet flat on the floor, hip-distance apart. On an inhalation, lift your arms overhead with palms facing each other and fingers pointing towards the ceiling. As you exhale, keep your back straight and press your weight through your heels to partially stand up from your chair until your legs are about 45 degrees. Hold here for about three to five bre-aths before slowly lowering back to your chair to return to the mountain pose.

Repeat steps two to four, twisting to the left for your spinal twist and using your left leg to start Warrior 2.

HIP CIRCLES

As the name suggests, seated hip circles involve moving your hips in a circular motion while sitting on your chair. It's similar to pelvic movements you would do from a standing position.

Sit on your chair with a straight spine and your hands on your thighs or knees. Begin making slow circular movements with your upper body at your hips in a clockwise rotation. As you continue to rotate, let your circles become larger. After at least five rotations, return to the center and repeat in a counter-clockwise rotation.

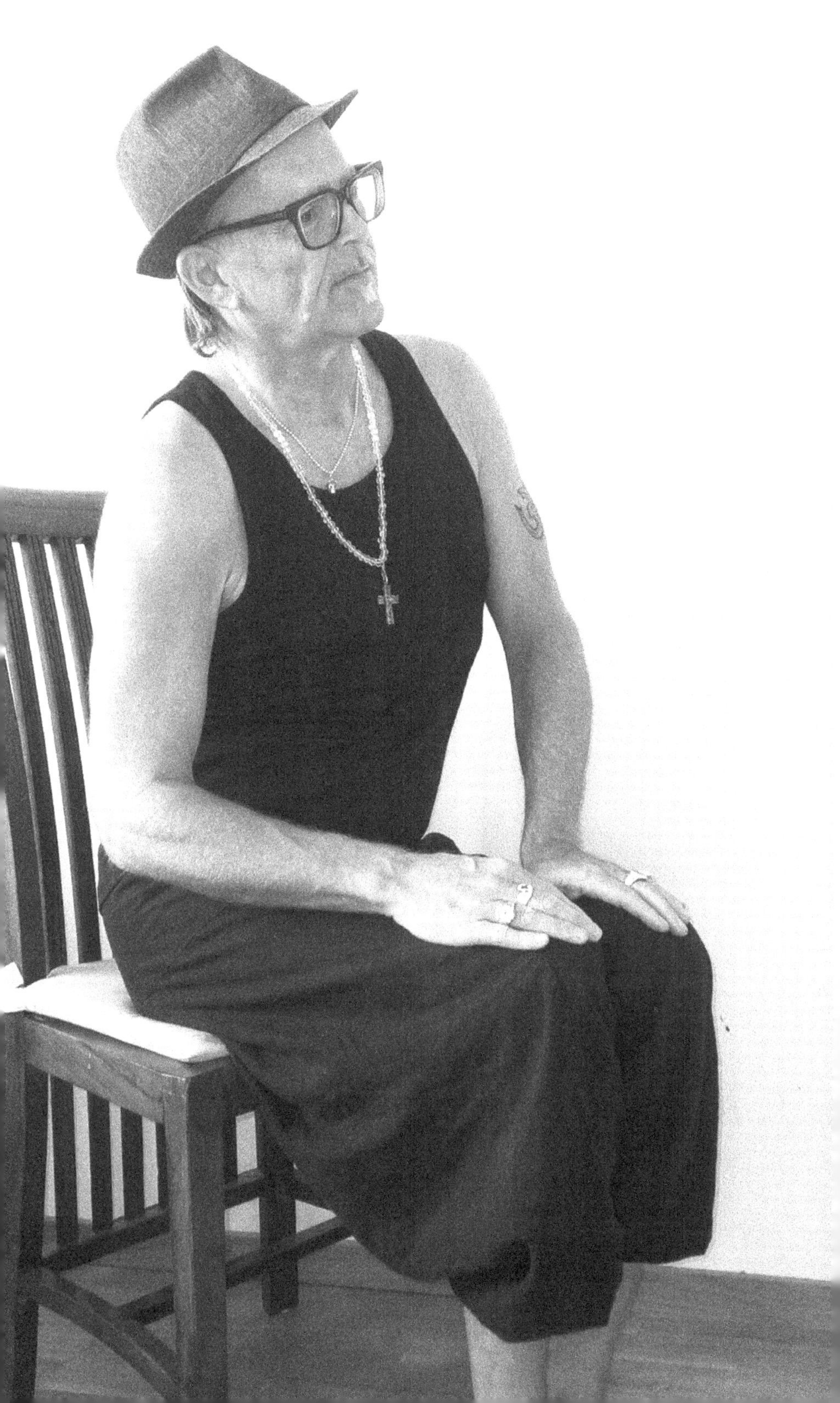

HALF-WIND RELEASE POSE

The wind release position is just as it sounds: it can help release gas built up in the abdomen. Stretching your hamstrings can also help alleviate stress and pain in your hips.

Sit on your chair with your legs about hip-width apart. Lift your right leg and grasp your fingers behind your knee to bring your leg closer to your chest. Hold for a few breaths, then release. Repeat on the other side.

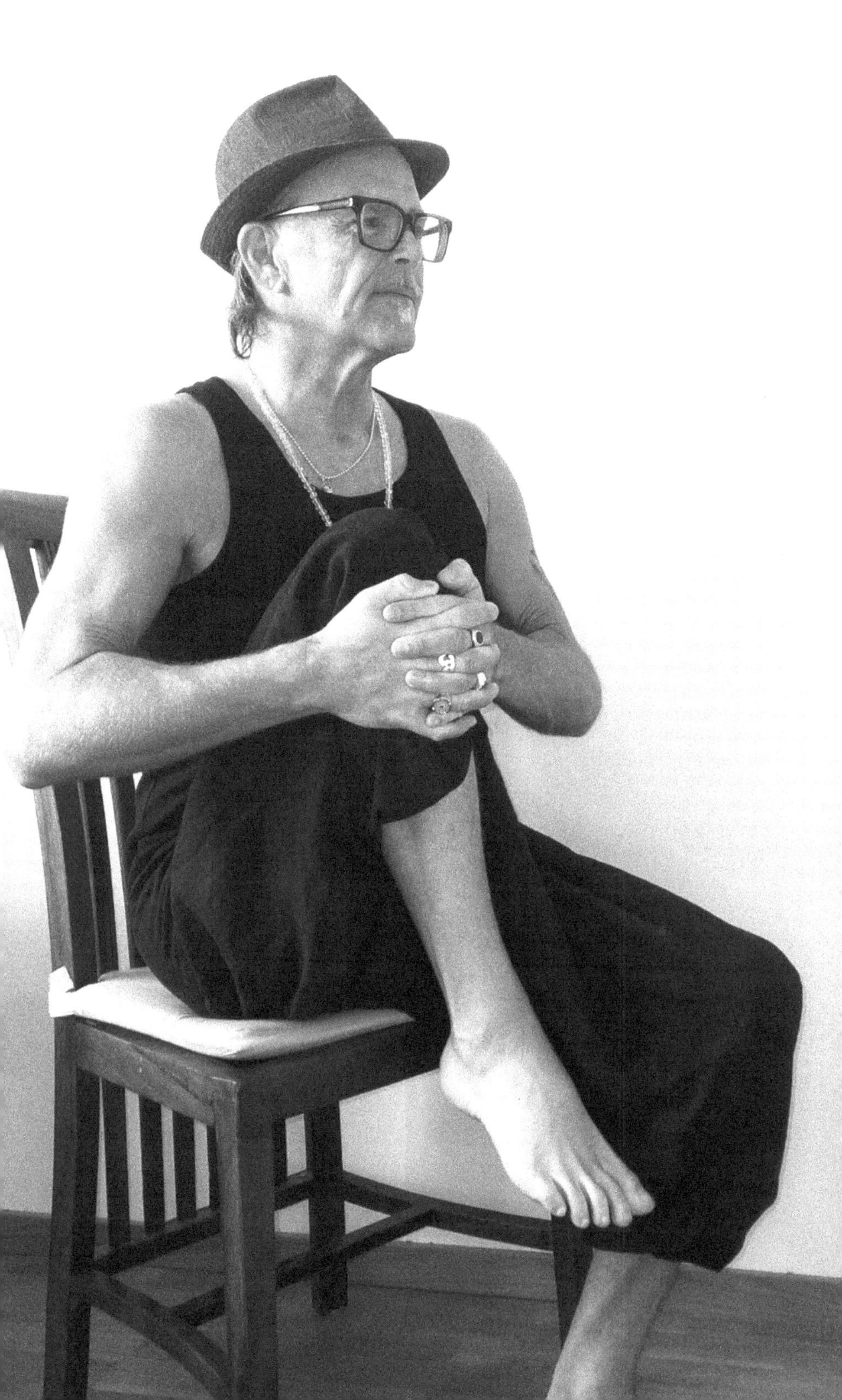

FLOW FOR SOFTER JOINTS 2

Start with hip circles by sitting upright on your chair with your feet on the floor and your hands resting on your knees or thighs. Imagine sitting on a giant clock and trying to move your hips to each number, making large circles in a clockwise rotation. As you continue to rotate, allow your circles to become more prominent. After five rotations, return to the center and repeat counterclockwise. After your last hip circle, return to a neutral sitting position to prepare for deep hip stretches.

Ensure your feet are flat on the floor and your legs are hip-width apart. Lift your right leg from the floor and bring your right knee towards your chest for a half-wind release pose.

Grasp your fingers behind your knee to pull your leg closer to your chest. Hold this position for a few breaths and feel a gentle stretch in your right hip. When ready, release and return your right foot to the floor.

Transition into pigeon pose by placing your right ankle over your left knee. If this feels comfortable, you can stay here. If you want a deeper stretch, gently lean forward from your hips. You should feel this in your right hip for a good stretch and balance challenge. After a few breaths in the pigeon, gently uncross your leg and return your foot to the floor.

Shift forward slightly on your chair to allow space for your feet to come together. Press the soles of your feet on your yoga block or chair and let your knees fall to the sides. Hold the bound angle for a few breaths.

Repeat steps two to four, focusing on your left side for half wind release pose and pigeon.

SHAKTI

This position helps us to open our hips, legs, and chest and strengthen our legs and shoulders. It also stretches the shoulder joint and chest muscles.

Sit on your chair in the mountain pose with a straight back and your hands resting on your thighs. On your inhale, open your legs to a wide stance, ensuring your knees are over your ankles and your toes point outward. Lift your arms overhead. Exhale and bend your elbows. Hold for a few moments.

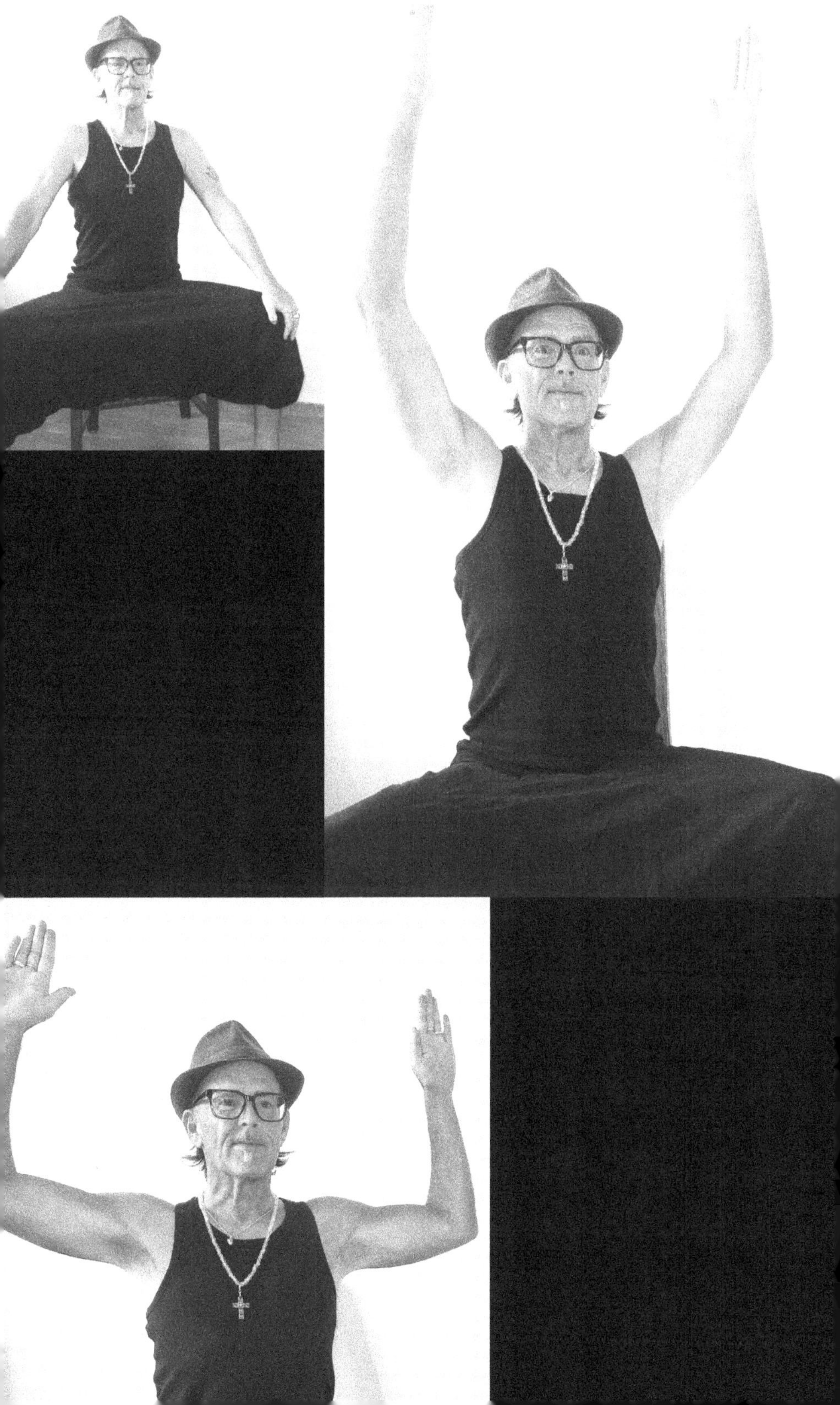

SHAKTI WITH SPINAL TWIST

This twisted position adds an extra level as your legs will be spread apart. This additional element will help stretch your hips as you twist.

Additionally, this position will help release any tension in the spine.

Sit on your chair in the mountain pose with a straight back and your hands resting on your thighs. On your inhale, open your legs to a wide stance, ensuring your knees are over your ankles and your toes point outward. Exhale as you twist your body to the right, gripping the back of your chair with your right arm and placing your left hand on the outside of your right thigh. Hold here for a few moments, then slowly come back. Repeat on the other side.

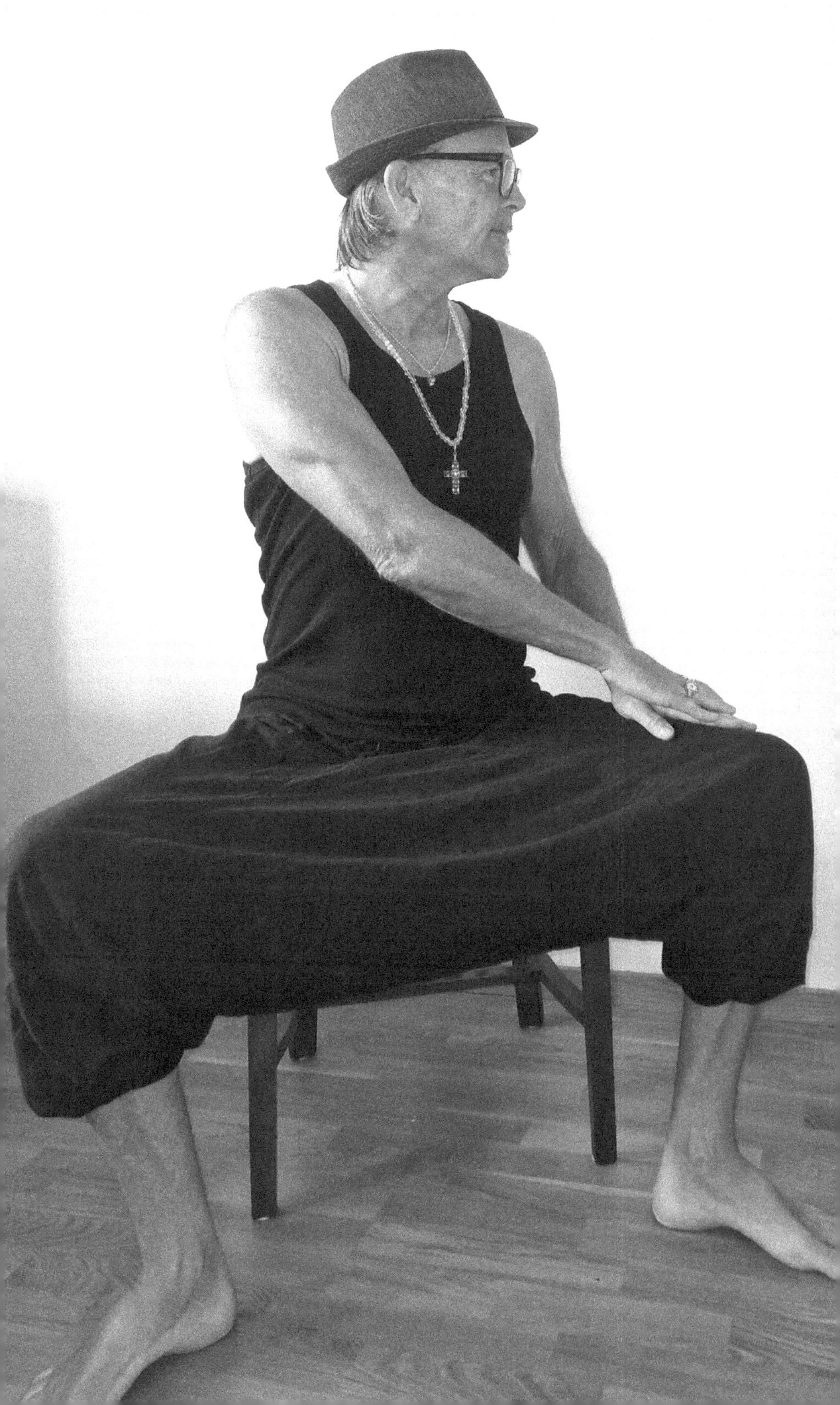

SHAKTI WITH SIDE BEND

Adding a side bend to Shakti will help lengthen your hip flexors and side muscles and release shoulder tension. This position will also help you open your chest muscles.

Sit on your chair in the mountain pose with a straight back and your hands resting on your thighs. On your inhale, open your legs to a wide stance, ensuring your knees are over your ankles and your toes point outward. Place your hands behind your head. Exhale as you lean to the right side, directing your right elbow toward the floor. Inhale to come back to the center. Repeat on the other side.

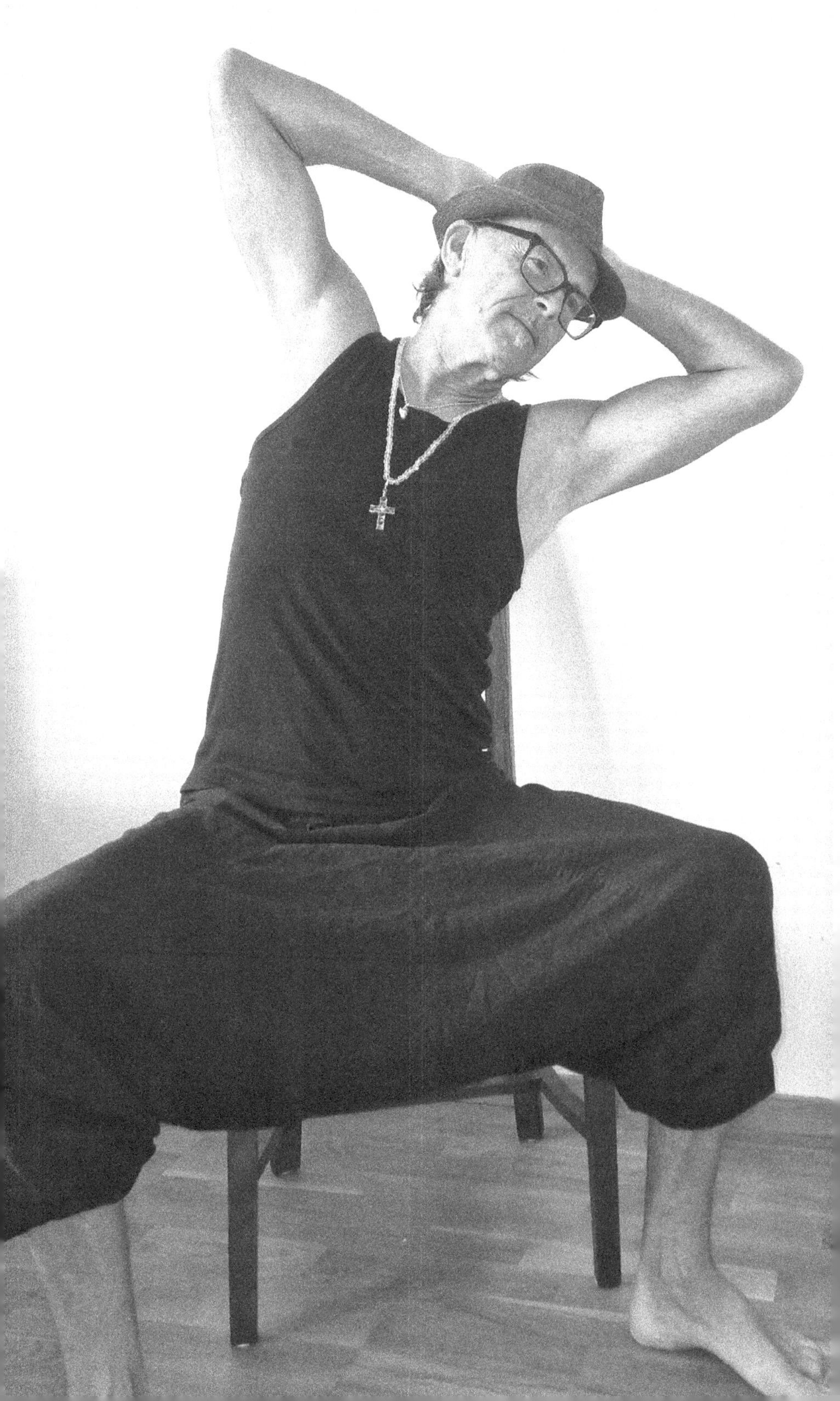

SHAKTI WITH FORWARD BEND

The position will stretch your hips, groin, inner thighs, and back while strengthening your shoulders, lower back, and knees. This movement is excellent for those who have diffi-culty bending forward due to stiffness, as it only requires the hands to rest on the thighs.

Sit on your chair with your legs wide apart and your toes pointing outward. With your hands on your inner thighs, inhale to engage your core muscles. Slowly lean forward until your spine is at a diagonal angle. Hold for a few moments, then slowly sit back up to an upright position.

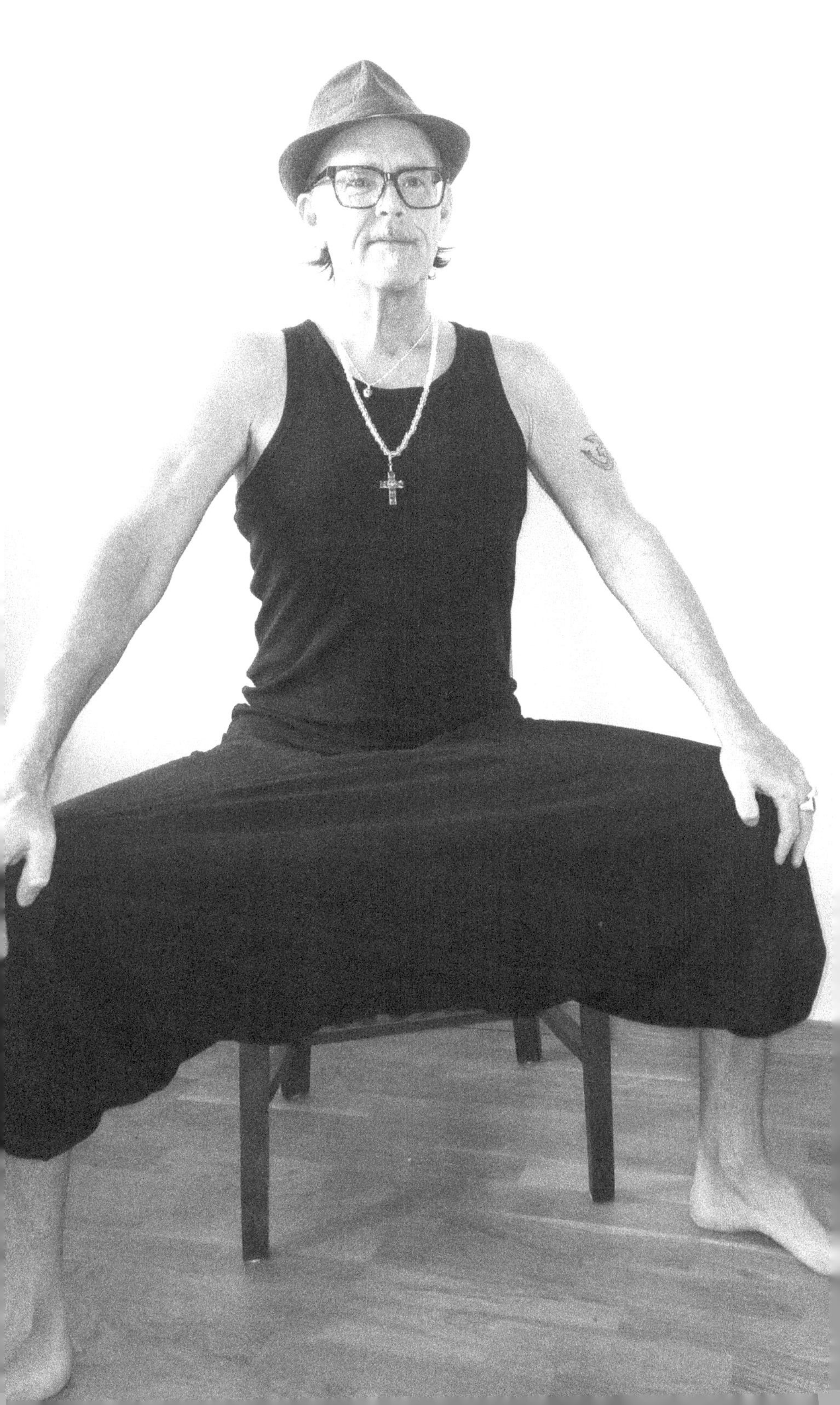

FLOW FOR SOFTER JOINTS 3

Begin by sitting on your chair in the mountain pose.

Then, enter Shakti: inhale to open your legs into a wide stance and lift your arms overhead. Exhale and bend your elbows. Hold briefly, then slowly lower your arms to the sides. Sit here for a few moments to experience your legs, shoulders, and chest stretch.

From shakti, transition into shakti with spinal twist by twisting your upper body to the right. Grip the back of your chair with your right arm and place your left hand outside your right thigh. Hold here for a few moments, then slowly twist back to the center and repeat on the other side.

From the spinal twist, move into shakti with a side bend by leaning to the right side, directing your right elbow towards the floor. Inhale to return to the center and repeat on the other side.

Finally, enter shakti with a forward bend by slowly leaning forward until your spine is diagonal. Hold for a few moments, then slowly sit back up to an upright position.

Repeat the entire flow a few times for full effect.

5

CHAIR YOGA

FOR FLEXIBILITY

Yoga is an ancient practice that promotes physical strength and balance and enhances mobility and flexibility. Yoga promotes profound mobility throughout the body by combining different poses (asanas), breathing exercises (pranayama), and meditation.

Stretching and elongating muscles and connective tissue: One of the most fundamental principles of yoga is the stretching of the body's muscles and connective tissue. Muscles are stretched in different directions by performing various yoga poses, promoting increased flexibility and mobility. Studies have shown that regular yoga can improve participants' muscle and joint mobility (Telles et al., 2016).

Improved muscle function and strength: Yoga involves passive stretches, active engagement, and strengthening of muscles. Yoga can increase joint mobility and stability by strengthening the muscles around the joints and improving their function (Broad et al., 2017).

Reduced muscle tension and stiffness: One of the most common causes of decreased mobility is muscle tension and stiffness. By performing various yoga poses and breathing exercises, practitioners can relax the muscles and reduce stress and stiffness, resulting in increased mobility and flexibility (Field, Diego, & Sanders, 2001).

Enhanced body posture and biomechanics: Yoga creates balance and symmetry by improving posture and movement patterns. By working with proper biomechanics and body mechanics during yoga poses, practitioners can increase mobility and reduce the risk of injury and pain (Wong et al., 2017).

Increased body awareness and presence: A central aspect of yoga is developing body awareness and presence. By being mindful of the body's movements and limits during yoga poses, practitioners can increase their mobility safely and sustainably (Wayne & Fuerst, 2013).

In summary, yoga offers an effective method for increasing body mobility through stretching, strengthening exercises, relaxation techniques, and improved body posture. By regularly practicing yoga, practitioners can experience various benefits for their mobility and flexibility, translating into increased comfort, freedom of movement, and overall well-being in daily life.

REFERENCES

Telles, S., Sharma, S. K., Yadav, A., & Singh, N. (2016). Immediate effect of three yoga breathing techniques on performance on a letter-cancellation task. Perceptual and Motor Skills, 122(1), 187-195.

Broad, W., Lin, Y., Majumdar, B., Chang, C. Y., Lee, S., Hsu, Y., ... & Cheng, W. (2017). Yoga's potential for promoting healthy aging: a narrative review. Journal of Aging and Physical Activity, 25(4), 1-10.

Field, T., Diego, M., & Sanders, C. (2001). Exercise is positively related to adolescents' relationships and academics. Adolescence, 36(141), 105.

Wong, A. Y., Parent, E. C., Dhillon, S. S., Prasad, N., & Kawchuk, G. N. (2017). Do participants with low back pain who respond to spinal manipulative therapy differ biomechanically from nonresponders, untreated controls or asymptomatic controls?. Spine, 42(24), 1909-1919.

Wayne, P. M., & Fuerst, M. L. (2013). The Harvard Medical School guide to yoga: 8 weeks to strength, awareness, and flexibility. Da Capo Lifelong Books.

INSTRUCTIONS BEFORE THE YOGA SESSION

Cleanse the nose with a neti pot (a nasal rinsing can with lukewarm water and salt) or nasal spray. Refrain from eating heavy food approximately 2–3 hours before. Preferably, be vegetarian. Do not drink caffeine. All of this calms the mind and gets the blood and prana moving in the body. Sit relaxed with a straight back.

HEAD CIRCLES

Sit on your chair with your hands resting on your thighs or knees and a straight back. Take a slow, deep breath in. Make a slow circle with your head in a clockwise direction on the exhale. Imagine your nose pointing at a clock. Start at 12 o'clock and circle your head around as if your nose is moving between the minutes and hours on the clock. After five rotations, change direction to circle your head counterclockwise, making sure to begin with a slow inhale.

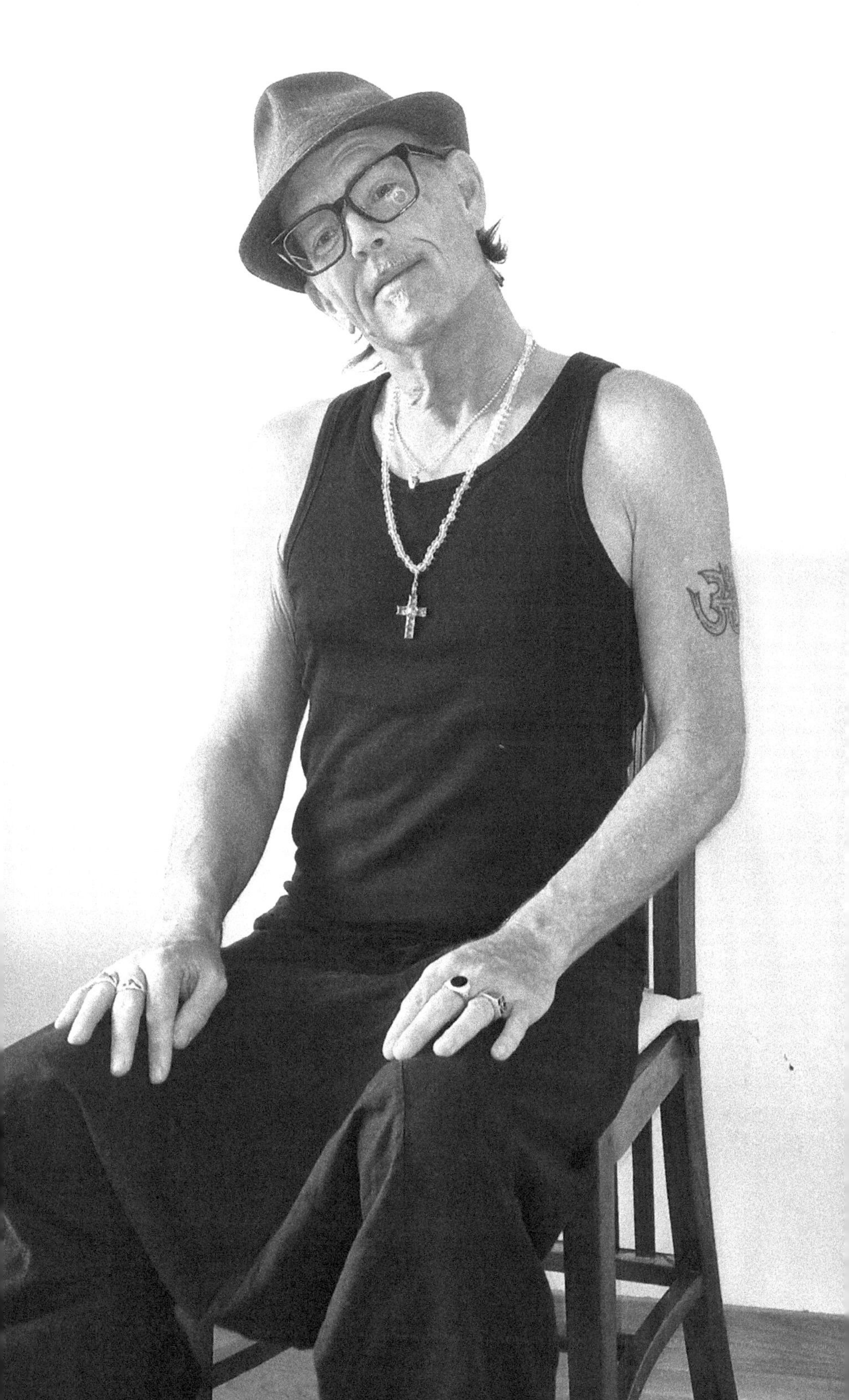

SHOULDER ROLLS

Our shoulders are another area where we tend to hold stress. Additionally, if you sleep on your side, you may tense one of your shoulders up to your ears (and you may not even realize it). Shoulder rolls help to restore the range of motion in your shoulder joints and muscles. Even without tense shoulders, it feels good to do them occasionally. Sit upright on your chair with your hands resting on your thighs or knees. Lift your shoulders towards your ears and roll them down to create a rotation. Continue with the same movement until you reach ten shoulder rolls, gradually making the rolls larger. Then, change direction and follow the same steps.

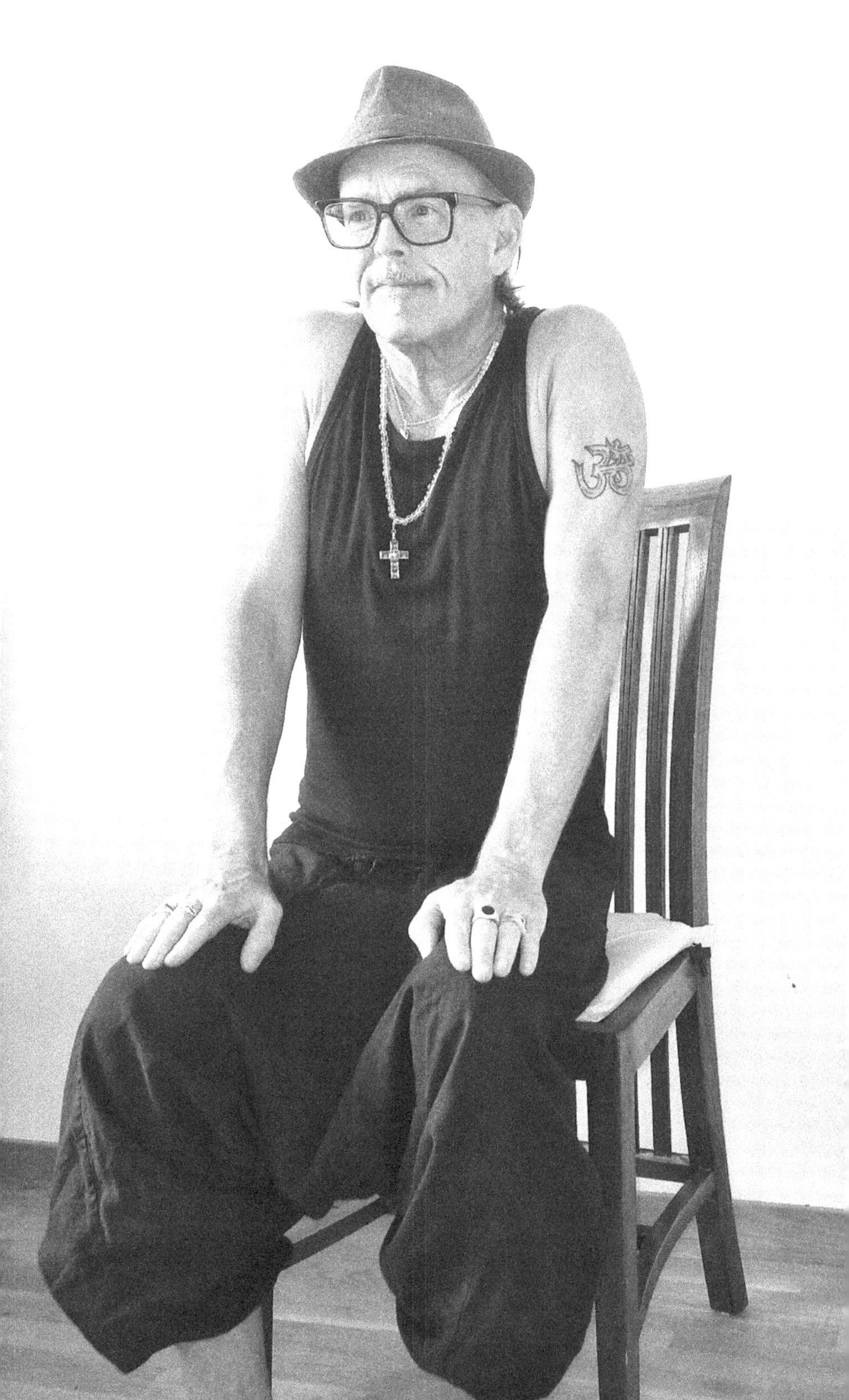

FLOW FOR INCREASED MOBILITY 1

Start with some head circles by sitting comfortably with your feet firmly on the floor and your hands resting on your thighs or knees with a straight back. Take a slow, deep breath. On the exhale, lower your chin to your chest and slowly roll your head clockwise in a large circle, then let it fall backward, then to the right, forward, and left. Do this a few times in both directions. Be careful with your movements to ensure it feels good in your neck. Lift your head back to a neutral position.

Move on to shoulder rolls by lifting your shoulders towards your ears, then roll them backward, down, and forward in a circular motion. Start with small rotations and gradually increase to larger ones, then change direction. It is an easy way to loosen stiff shoulder joints. After your final shoulder roll, let your shoulders relax and place your arms beside you. Inhale and lift your left arm overhead with the palm facing inward for a side stretch.

Place your right hand beside the chair for stability. Exhale as you bend to the right, creating a "C" shape. You'll feel a nice stretch along your left side. After a few breaths, return to the center and lower your left arm to prepare for a spinal twist.

Adjust your arms by placing your left hand on your right knee and your right hand on the back of the chair. Take a deep breath in and, as you exhale, twist your upper body to the right. Ensure your spine remains straight as you hold for a few breaths. Inhale to come back to the center for a hamstring stretch.

137

Move your buttocks close to the edge of the chair. Extend your left leg straight forward with the toes pointing towards the ceiling. Inhale and bend forward to feel the stretch in your left hamstring. Stretch your hands towards your left foot resting on the shin. Listen to your body and stretch as far as feels good. After a few breaths, relax and return to the center.

Repeat steps four to six on the right side.

THE EAGLE

Sit on your chair in the mountain pose. Cross your right leg over your left foot and tuck your right foot behind your left calf if you can. If this isn't possible, keep your legs in the mountain position with feet hip-width apart. Hug yourself by crossing your arms over your chest and touching the opposite shoulders with your right arm on top. If you can, lift the backs of your hands to meet in front of your face. If you can go further, tuck your left hand so that your fingers touch your right palm. Lift your elbows to deepen the stretch and hold for a few breaths with a straight spine. Release and switch sides.

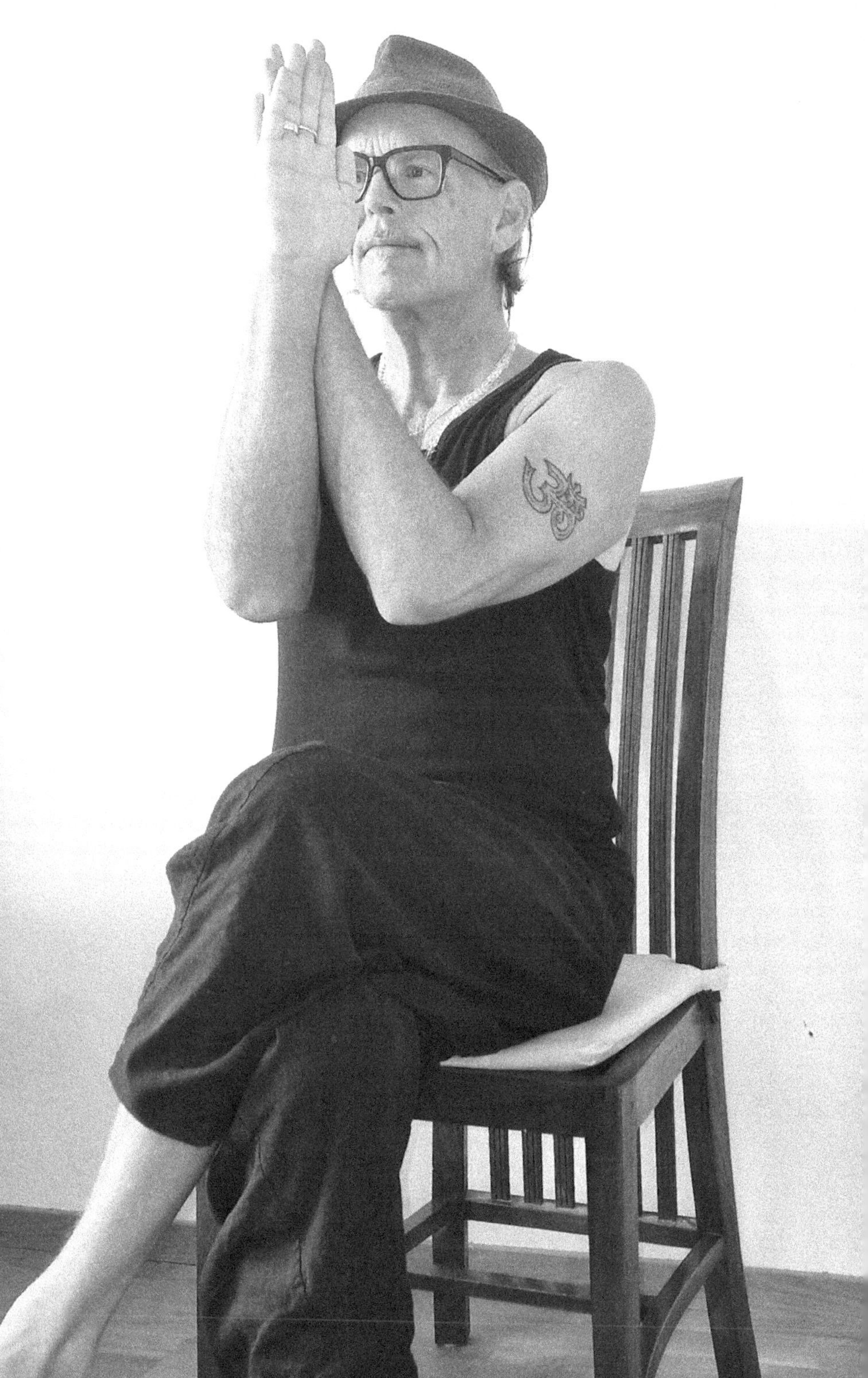

FLOW FOR INCREASED MOBILITY 2

Start by sitting comfortably on your chair, with your feet grounded on the floor, shoulder-width apart, and hands resting on your thighs or knees. Sit up and roll your shoulders back, opening your chest. Inhale to engage your core and lift your spine. As you exhale, place one hand on your heart and the other on your abdomen, and imagine your body rooting into the ground.

Continue with shoulder rolls by lifting your shoulders towards your ears, then rolling them backward, down, and forward in a circular motion. Start with small rotations and gradually increase to larger ones, then change direction. Inhale and stretch your arms towards the sky, lengthening your spine. As you exhale, bend forward from your hips, letting your hands rest on your shins, ankles, or the floor, depending on your flexibility. Let your head hang down for a few breaths, feeling the gentle stretch in your back.

When you're ready, roll up your body to the mountain pose. Scoot your buttocks close to the front edge of the chair. Extend your left leg straight forward with the toes pointing towards the ceiling. Inhale and bend forward to feel the stretch in your left hamstring. Stretch your hands towards your left foot resting on the shin. After a few breaths, relax and return to the center.

Enter the eagle pose by crossing your arms over your chest and touching the opposite shoulders with your right arm on top. Lift the backs of your hands to meet in front of your face. If you want to go further, tuck your left hand so that your fingers touch your right palm. Lift your elbows to deepen the stretch and hold here for a few breaths, maintaining your posture. Relax your arms and let them rest in your lap before moving into a spinal twist.

Inhale as you place your left hand on your right knee and your right hand on the back of your chair. As you exhale, twist your torso to the right, looking over your right shoulder. Take deep breaths here for a few moments, then inhale to return to the center.

Repeat steps two to five, focusing on your left side for the eagle and spinal twist.

FLOW FOR INCREASED MOBILITY 3

Start by sitting comfortably on your chair, with your feet firmly on the floor, as we move through a flow similar to a sun salutation.

Begin in the mountain pose with your knees directly over your ankles, hip-width apart. Please take a deep breath, lift your arms overhead, and stretch them towards the sky. Exhale into a prayer position as you bring your hands to your heart center.

Maintain this hand position as you fold into a forward bend by hinging at your hips and rounding your back. Release your hands towards your feet. Inhale and roll up, imagining your vertebrae stacking on each other with your head coming last. Finally, roll your shoulders so they draw away from your ears, and let your hands rest on your thighs.

Place your hands on your thighs for the cat pose. Inhale, arch your back, and roll down your shoulders, lifting your chest and looking upward. Exhale, round your back, and let your shoulders and head come forward. Continue flowing between these two positions several times, linking your breath with the movement. Return to a neutral spine after your final round of the cat pose.

Ensure your feet are flat on the floor and your legs are hip-width apart. Lift your right leg from the floor and bring your right knee towards your chest for a half-wind relea-se pose. Clasp your fingers behind your knee to draw your leg closer to your chest. Hold this position for a few breaths, feeling a gentle stretch in your right hip. When ready, release and return your right foot to the floor before switching sides.

Slide to the edge of your chair, keeping your feet flat on the floor, hip-width apart for the reverse chair pose. Inhale, lift your arms overhead with palms facing each other and fingers pointing towards the ceiling. Keep your spine straight as you exhale, and press your weight through your heels to partially stand up from your chair until your legs are about 45 degre-es. Hold here for about three to five breaths before slowly lowering back to your chair to return to the mountain pose.

Lift your arms again to repeat the reverse chair pose, pres-sing through your heels. After three to five breaths this time, straighten your spine to standing. As you stand, turn towards your chair for a variation of the mountain pose. Bend your torso towards the chair seat and take a few steps forward until your body forms an excellent "V" shape, with your hips at the highest point. Press your palms against the chair, draw in your belly, and push your heels towards the floor for a deep stretch through your shoulders and back. Hold this position briefly before slowly sliding back to your chair to conclude your routine.

6

CHAIR YOGA

FOR STRENGTH

Yoga is not only a practice for relaxation and flexibility; it can also be a powerful method for increasing body strength. By performing various yoga poses and exercises, practitioners can develop muscle strength and endurance in a sustainable and functional way.

Muscle Activation and Engagement: One of the fundamental principles of yoga is to use the body's weight and resistance to activate and strengthen the muscles. Various yoga poses, such as plank, warrior, and boat poses, engage different muscle groups in the body, including the core muscles, arms, legs, and back. Studies have shown that yoga can effectively increase muscle strength and improve muscle function in participants (Tran et al., 2018).

Strength Training through Isometric and Eccentric Loading: Many yoga poses involve holding a position for an extended period, creating isometric loading in the muscles. For example, keeping the plank or warrior pose requires the muscles to work hard to maintain the position, increasing strength and muscle endurance over time. Additionally, some yoga poses, especially those involving downward movements like Chaturanga Dandasana (cobra pose), involve eccentric loading, which can help increase muscle strength and reduce the risk of injuries (Zuhl & Kravitz, 2012).

Improved Body Posture and Stability: Yoga focuses on building strength in individual muscle groups and creating balance and stability throughout the body. By strengthening the core muscles and improving body posture, yoga can help prevent injuries and enhance performance in other physical activities and sports (Hagen et al., 2015).

Integration of Breath and Strength: A unique feature of yoga is the integration of breathing techniques (pranayamas) with physical exercises. By coordinating breathing with movements, practitioners can increase their energy, focus, and strength during practice. Studies have shown that deep and mindful breathing can help increase muscle strength and endurance and reduce fatigue and stress during exercise (Marshall et al., 2018).

Injury Prevention and Promotion of Recovery: By strengthening the muscles and improving the body's stability and flexibility, yoga can also help prevent injuries and promote faster recovery after exercise or physical exertion (Gong et al., 2015).

Summary: By regularly practicing yoga, practitioners can experience various benefits for their strength, which can translate into improved performance, increased muscle endurance, and reduced risk of injuries in daily life and during other physical activities.

REFERENCES

Tran, M. D., Holly, R. G., Lashbrook, J., & Amsterdam, E. A. (2018). Effects of Hatha yoga practice on the health-related aspects of physical fitness. Preventive cardiology, 4(4), 165-170.

Zuhl, M., & Kravitz, L. (2012). Hiit vs. continuous endurance training: battle of the aerobic titans. IDEA Fitness Journal, 9(1), 1-8.

Hagen, M., Macmillan, F., Lutz, N., & Stanhope, J. (2015). Yoga for military veterans with chronic low back pain: A randomized clinical trial. American journal of preventive medicine, 49(6), 822-831.

Marshall, M., Berstein, K., & Wu, S. (2018). The effects of deep breathing exercises and diaphragmatic breathing exercises in treating musculoskeletal dysfunction. International Journal of Yoga and Physical Therapy, 1(1), 14-20.

Gong, H., Ni, C. X., Liu, Y. Z., Zhang, Y., Su, W. J., Lian, Y. J., ... & Jiang, C. L. (2015). Yoga for prenatal depression: a systematic review and meta-analysis. BMC psychiatry, 15(1), 14.

INSTRUCTIONS BEFORE THE YOGA SESSION

Cleanse the nose with a neti pot (a nasal rinsing can with lukewarm water and salt) or nasal spray. Refrain from eating heavy food approximately 2-3 hours before. Preferably, be vegetarian. Do not drink caffeine. All of this calms the mind and gets the blood and prana moving in the body. Sit relaxed with a straight back.

SINGLE LEG BOAT

In the first variation, you lift one leg and hold it in position. Start sitting on your chair in a mountain pose with a straight back. Your sitting bones should be near the edge of the chair, but ensure that your body feels stable and comfortable. Lift your right leg and clasp your fingers behind your knee. En-gage your core as you hold the pose and avoid rounding your back. Hold for about 30 seconds, then lower to switch legs. Repeat three times with each leg lifted.

Helpful tip: Use a yoga block or a rolled-up pillow if you need extra support under your foot.

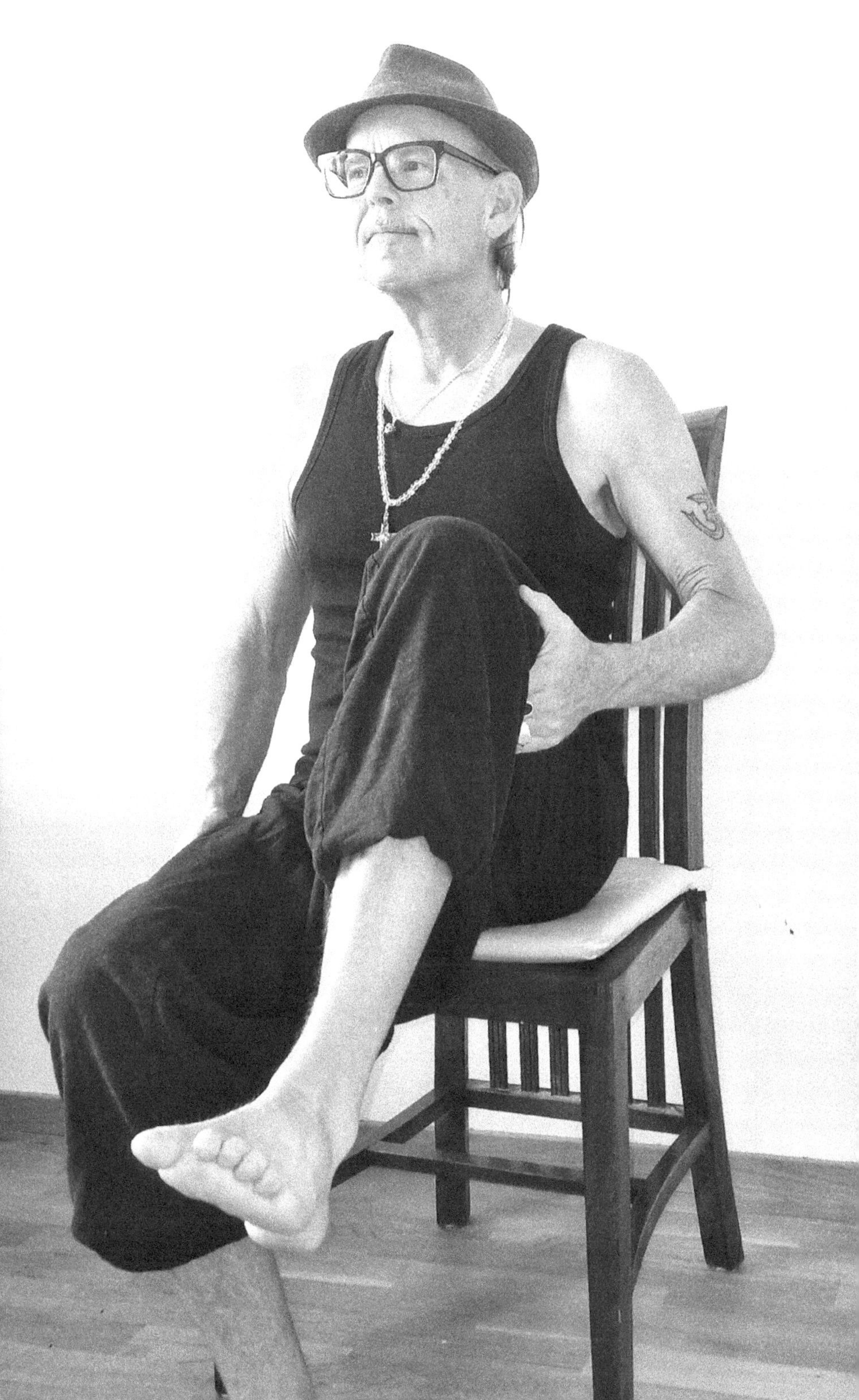

SINGLE-LEG BOAT WITH ONE ARM

You'll lift your right leg with a bent knee and extend your right arm out for this variation. Ensure you don't round your back while holding the position, and grab a yoga block or rolled-up pillow if you need support under your foot on the floor.

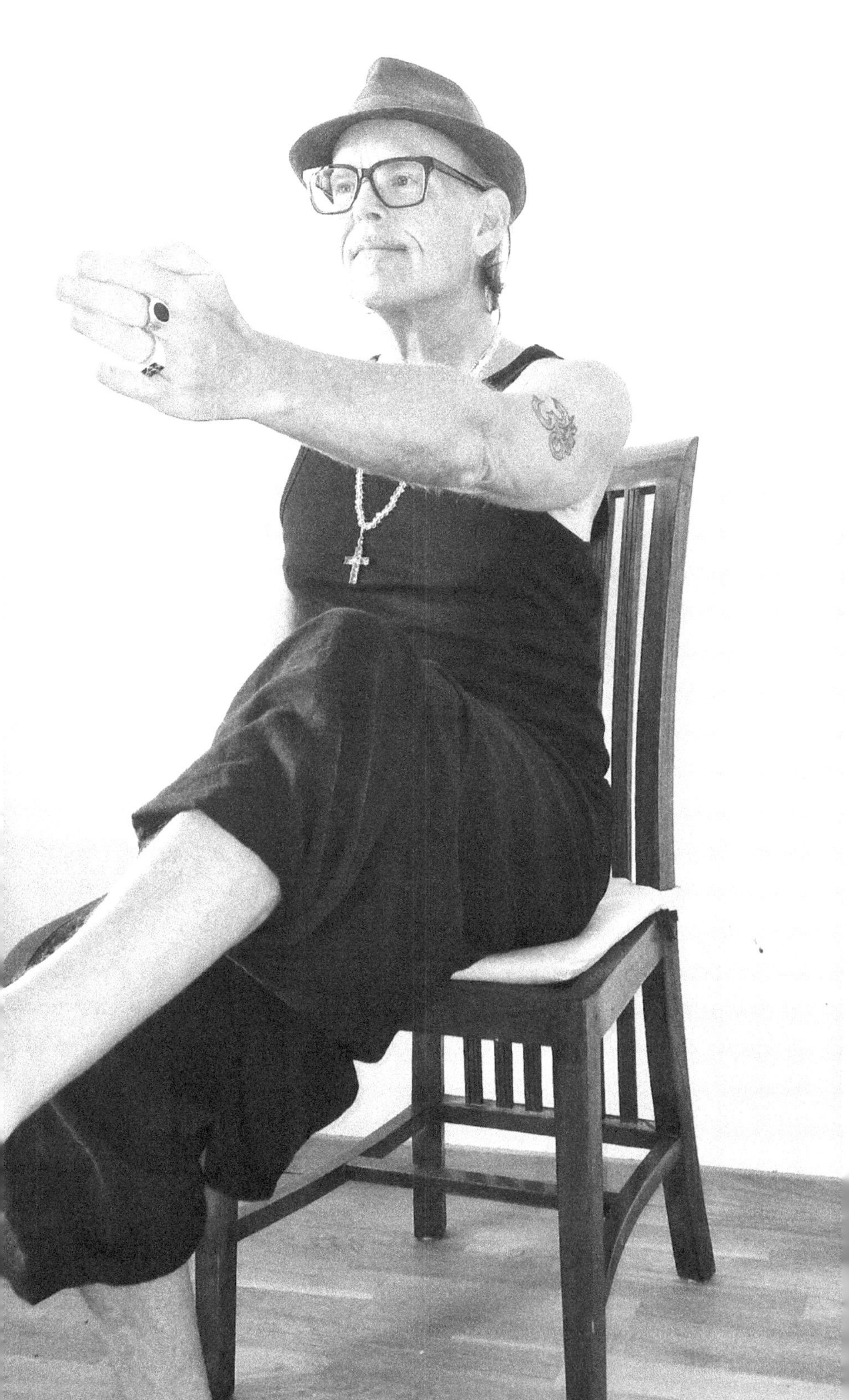

DOUBLE LEG BOAT

In this variation, follow the instructions above, except this time, you'll lift both legs and hold the backs of your thighs with each hand.

SEATED BOAT

You'll hold your legs in the air and your arms forward for the fully seated boat. It is the most challenging way to perform the boat pose, so don't give up if you don't get it right the first time.

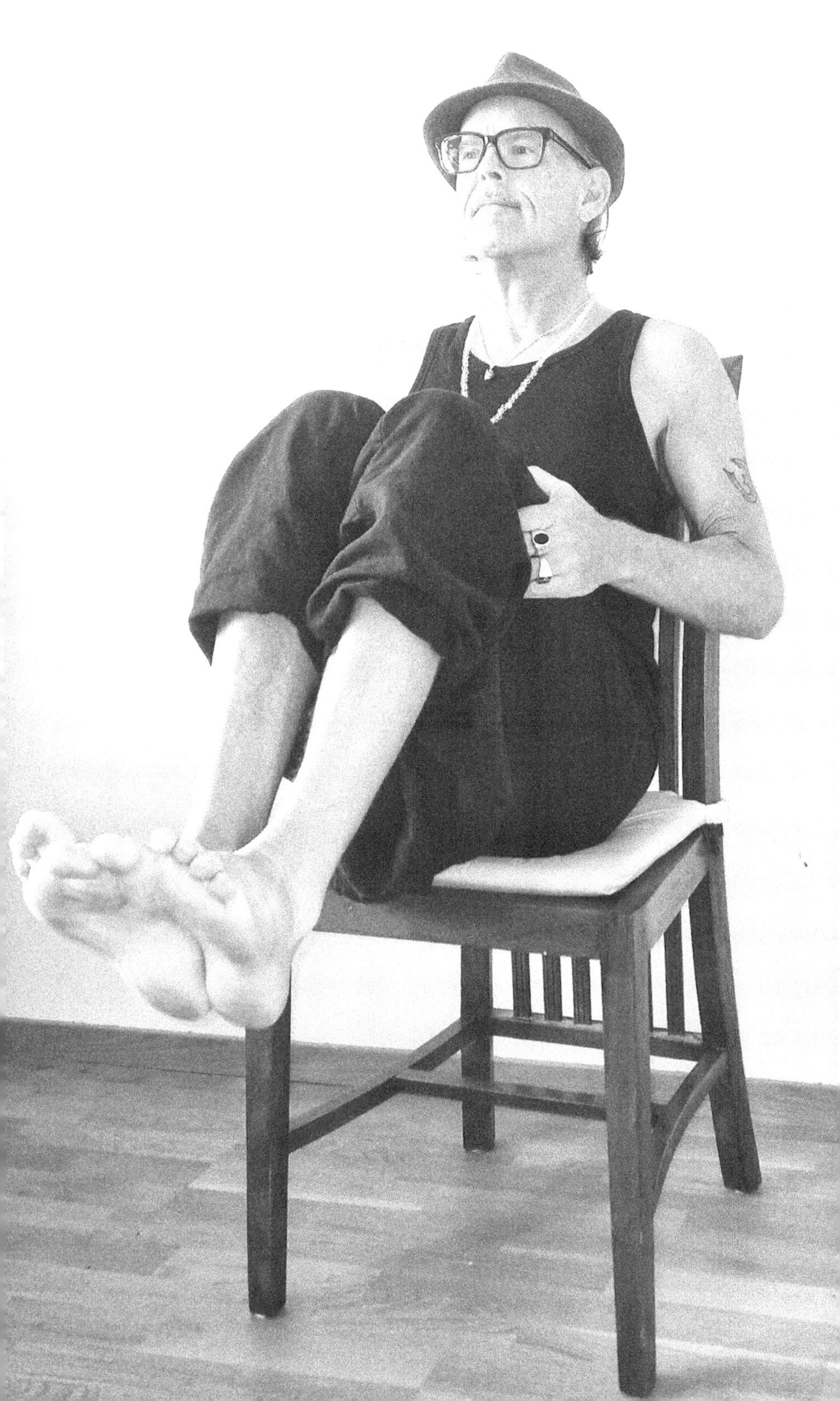

HIGH LUNGE

The high lunge with a chair will help support your leg so you can comfortably perform the pose. This position is excellent for building strength in your hips, thighs, and calf muscles, which can improve your stability. It also helps stretch your hip flexors, which can become stiff from prolonged sitting.

Begin by sitting in a mountain pose on your chair. Bring your right leg to the side of your chair as you twist your torso. Use the chair for support, and straighten your back leg with your toes curled under you. Rest your left hand on your leg. As you hold the position, engage your core muscles to find balance. If you feel stable, lift your arms overhead and hold. When you're ready, lower your arms if extended and bring in your left leg. Switch sides and follow the same steps.

For an extra challenge, place your foot on the seat of the chair and your hands on your hips. It will genuinely stretch and build muscles in your hip flexors.

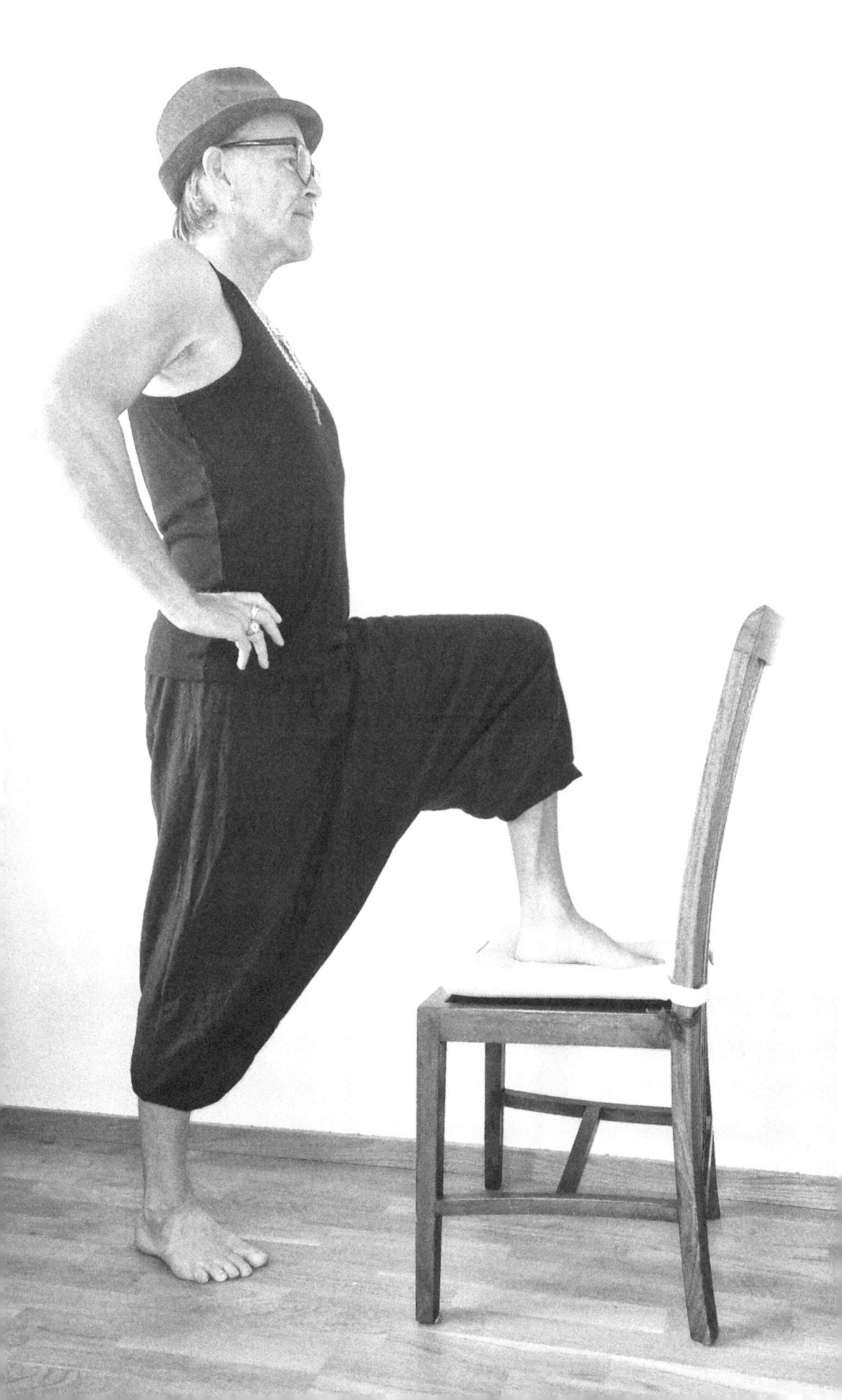

CAMEL

Sit on your chair in a mountain pose with your sitting bones near the front edge of the chair. Roll your shoulders away from your ears and place your hands on your lower back with your elbows pointing behind you. Gently lean your upper back to create a curve. If you can, lift your head towards the ceiling. Take a few breaths before returning to the starting position.

Repeat five times.

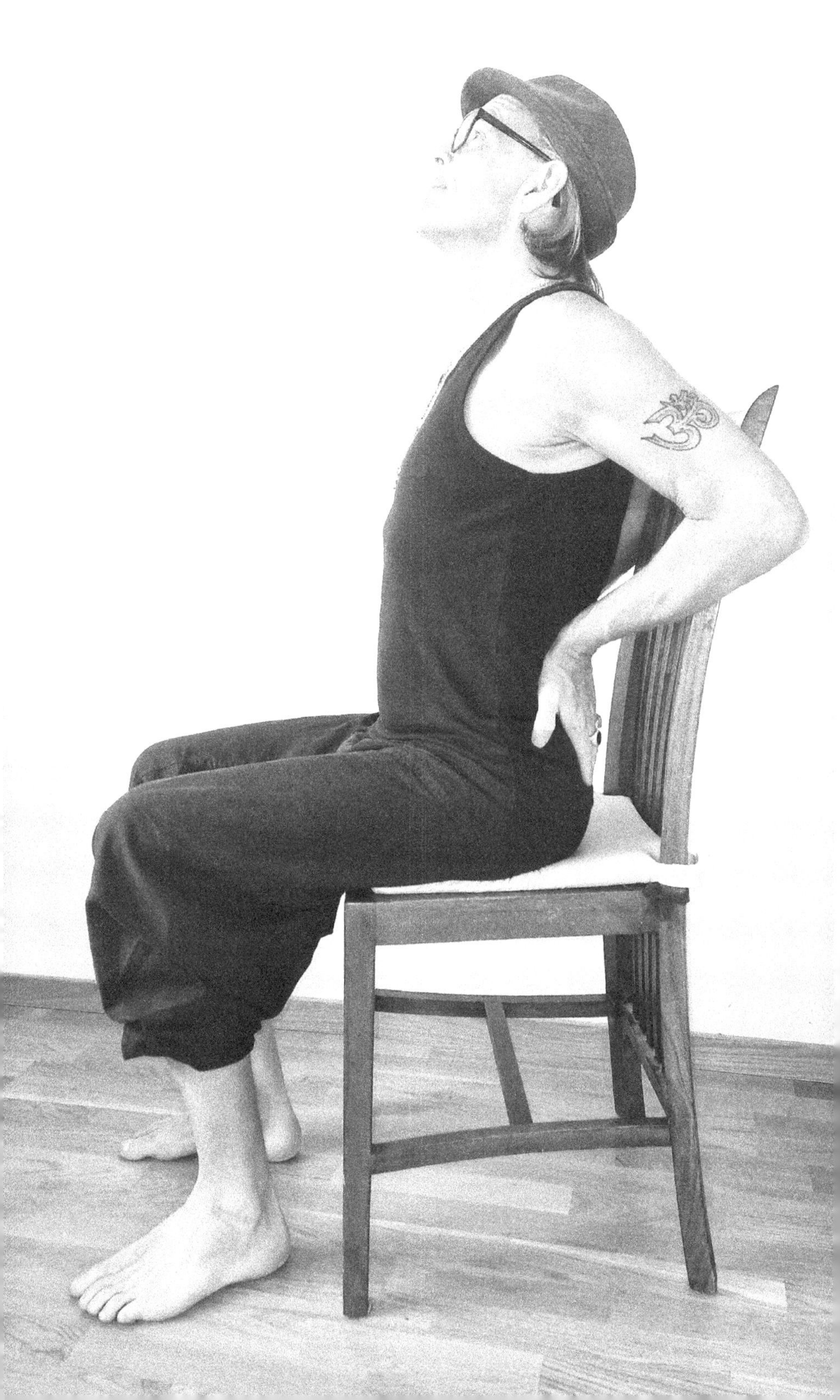

STRENGTH BUILDING FLOW 1

*Start sitting upright on the edge of your chair with your feet
flat on the floor. Get into camel pose: roll your shoulders
away from your ears and place your palms on your lower
back, fingers pointing down and elbows pointing behind you.
As you inhale, gently press your hips forward and arch your
back, lifting your chest towards the ceiling. You should feel the
stretch in your chest. Then, return to a neutral seated position.*

*Move into the eagle pose by crossing your arms over your
chest and touching the opposite shoulders with your right arm
on top. Lift the backs of your hands to meet each other in front
of your face. If you want to go further, bring your left hand so
your fingers touch your right palm. Lift your elbows to deepen
the stretch and hold here for a few breaths with maintained
posture. Slowly unroll your arms and let them rest on your
lap. You can also add your lower body to this exercise by crossing your right leg over your left and bringing your right foot
behind your left calf.*

*From the mountain pose, bring your right leg to the side of
your chair as you twist your torso 90 degrees to the right. Place your palms on the chair's seat for support and straighten
your back leg with your toes curled under you. Keep a straight
back and engage your core muscles to find balance. If you're
ready for the challenge, lift your arms overhead, palms facing
each other. After a few breaths, return to the center and re-*

peat the exercise on your left side. Glide forward to the front edge of your chair for a single-leg boat.

When you feel stable, lean back slightly, lift your right leg, and clasp your fingers behind your knee. Engage your core as you hold the position and avoid rounding your back. Hold here for three long breaths before lowering your leg and switching sides. Aim to complete five repetitions. After your final repetition, adjust yourself on your chair to ensure space for your feet to come together for a bound-angle pose.

Place the soles of your feet on your yoga block and let your knees fall to the sides. Hold for a couple of breaths. Gently return to a neutral seated position for a standing mountain pose.

Stand up from your chair and turn so you're facing the chair. Bend your torso towards the chair seat and take a few steps forward until your body forms an excellent "V" shape, with your hips at the highest point. Press your palms against the chair, draw in your belly, and push your hips back. Your head should be in line with your arms. On your final inhale, slowly roll up to a standing position.

Repeat the flow two to three more times to build strength and endurance.

TWISTED CHAIR

The twisted chair is another excellent pose for mobilizing your spine while strengthening your ankles, thighs, hip flexors, and glutes.

Sit on your chair with your feet together. Squeeze your knees together to activate your inner thigh muscles. Bring your hands together in a prayer position in the center of your chest. As you bend at your hips, twist your torso to the right so your elbow points towards the ceiling. Place your left elbow on the outside of your right knee. Roll your right shoulder back and look up towards the ceiling. Hold for five breaths, then return to the starting position. Switch sides. As you build strength in this exercise, you should be able to lift your support a few centimeters off the chair.

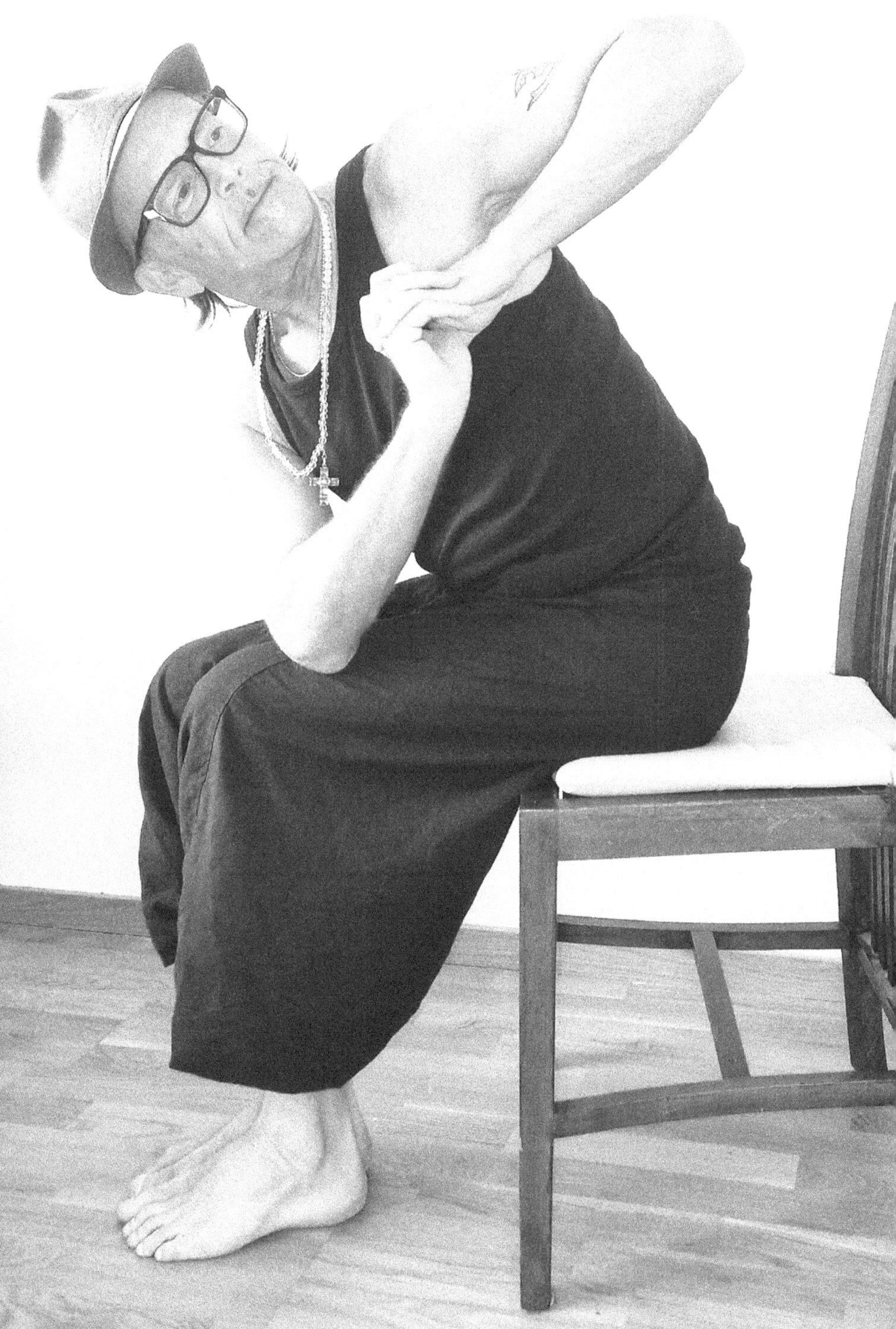

UPWARD PLANK

This is an excellent full-body exercise because it builds strength in your core, shoulders, arms, and legs.

Sit on the edge of your chair with your feet flat on the floor. Place your palms on the sides of your chair with your fingers pointing forward. As you inhale, gently press your hips upwards to create a straight line from your shoulders to your heels. Activate your thigh muscles to help support your legs. Remember to keep your neck in line with your spine and look up. Hold here for five breaths before lowering down and resting.

UPWARD PLANK WITH LEG LIFT

To further increase the challenge, lift one leg off the floor and hold for five breaths before switching legs.

PLANK WITH BENT KNEES

Plank pose is challenging for most of us! If you find it difficult to extend your legs forward, keep your feet flat on the floor and bend your knees to 45 degrees. Engage your core and hold the plank.

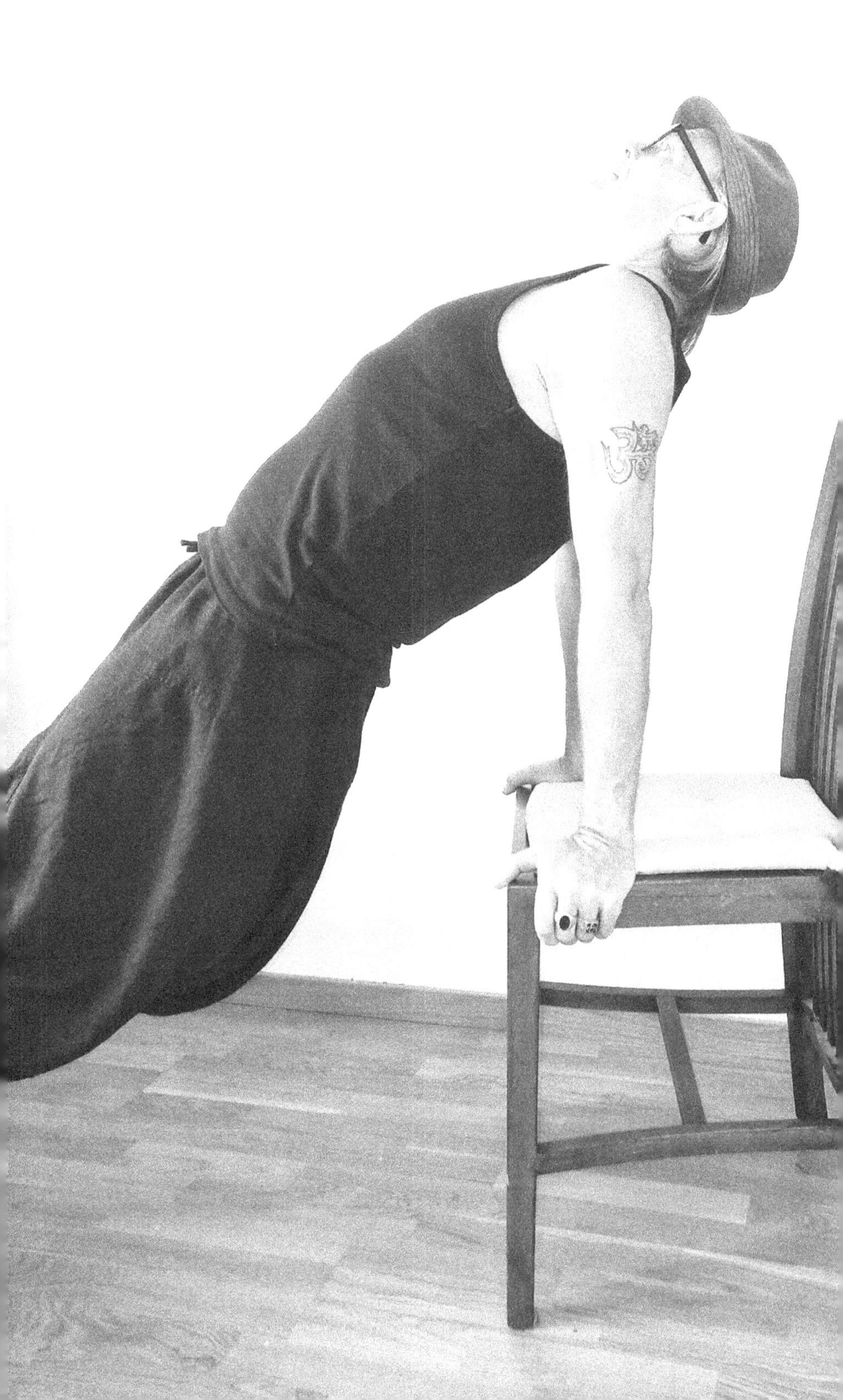

RAGDOLL

Ragdoll is excellent for releasing leg, hips, and back tension to improve your overall flexibility.

Stand in front of your chair with your feet hip-width apart. Let your fingertips lead as you slowly roll forward and bend at the hips. Bring your arms together overhead and grab your elbows. Let your head hang between your arms. Rock gently from side to side in a soft motion. When you're ready, slowly roll back up. If you find it challenging to hang freely, rest your forearms on the chair seat.

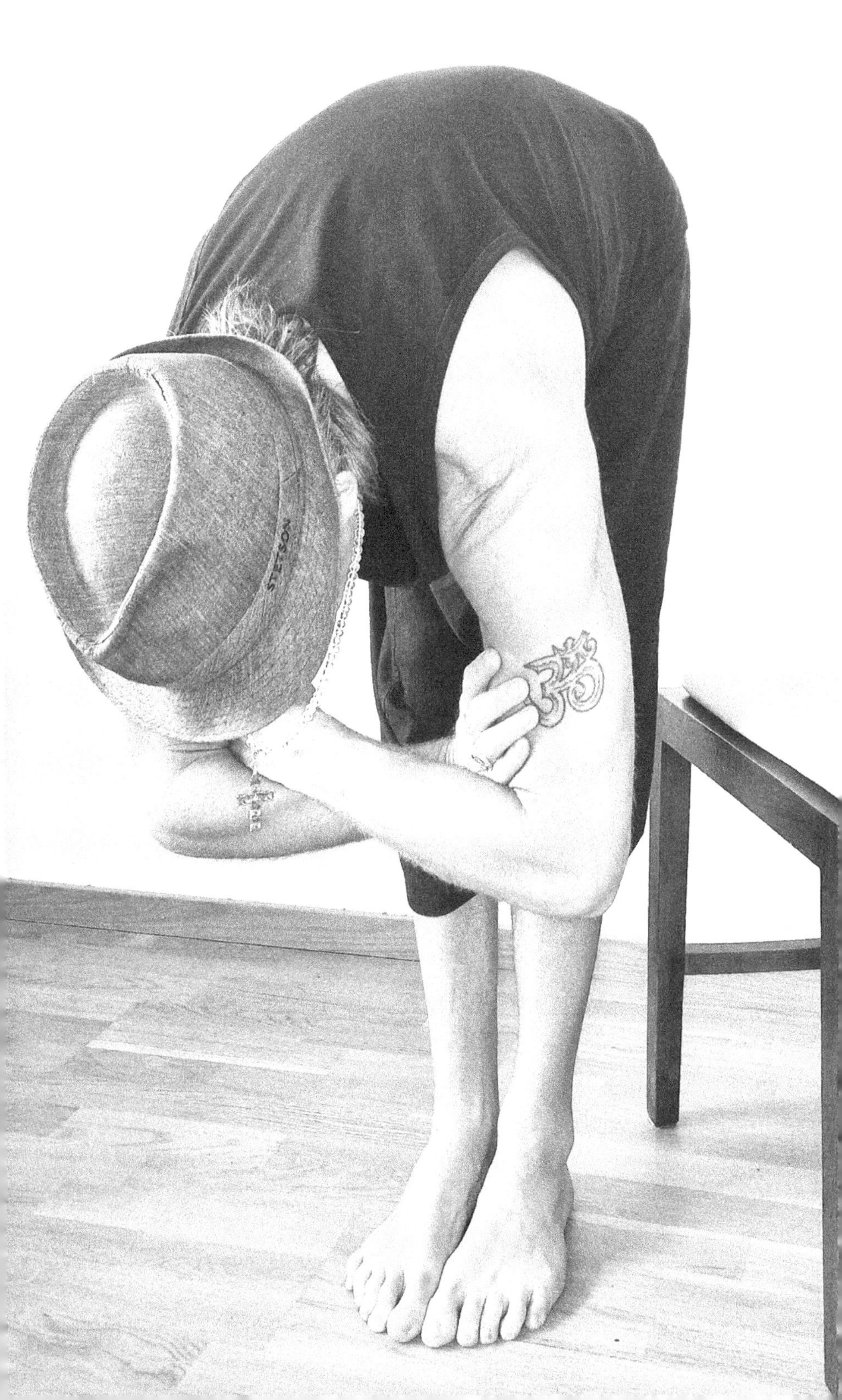
STETSON

STRENGTH BUILDING FLOW 2

Start this strength training sequence with the reverse chair. Glide to the edge of your chair and keep your feet flat on the floor a hip distance apart. On an inhale, lift your arms overhead with palms facing each other and fingers poin- ting towards the ceiling. Then, as you exhale, keep your back straight and press the weight through your heels to partially stand up from the chair until your legs reach about 45 de- grees. Hold here for about three to five breaths before slowly lowering back to your chair to return to mountain pose and prepare for any boat pose.

Choose the boat variation you want to perform. When you feel stable, lean back slightly and lift one or both legs with fing- ers locked behind the knee. Engage your core as you hold the position and avoid rounding your back. If you're ready for an extra challenge, unlock your fingers and lift your arms. Hold three breaths before lowering one or both legs and returning to the mountain pose.

Sit on the front edge of your chair. Place your palms on the seat just behind your buttocks, with your knuckles facing the front, for an upward plank. Extend both legs diagonally before you, with your toes pointing towards the ceiling. By pressing into your hands and engaging your core, lift your buttocks off the chair to create a straight line with your body. Hold two to three breaths before slowly lowering back to your chair.

Return to mountain pose but with your feet together for the twisted chair.

Squeeze your knees together to activate your inner thigh muscles as you bring your hands to a prayer position in the center of your chest. Then, as you bend at the hips, twist your torso to the right so your right elbow points towards the ceiling and your left elbow rests outside your right knee. Make sure not to collapse your shoulders but to roll them back to create a straight line from elbow to elbow. Hold for five breaths before twisting back to center.

To conclude the flow, stand up from your chair with your feet hip-width apart. Let your fingertips lead as you slowly roll forward, bending at the hips until you reach a comfortable position. Get into a ragdoll, bend your arms overhead, grab your elbows, and let your head hang between your arms. Rock gently from side to side to help stretch your back and leg muscles. When you're ready, slowly roll back up. Repeat all steps with the seated twisted chair to the left.

EXTENDED SIDE ANGLE OR TWISTED CHAIR

Seated extended side angle can help relieve stiffness in your shoulders, back, and side while building strength in your hips and thigh muscles. Begin in mountain pose. Open your right leg to the side outside of your chair, making sure your knee is stacked over your ankle. Then, extend your left leg to the side with your toes pointing forward. Rest your right forearm on your right leg as you extend your left arm overhead. If you can, twist your head to face your extended arm. Exit the position by lowering your left arm and sitting back up. Repeat on the other side.

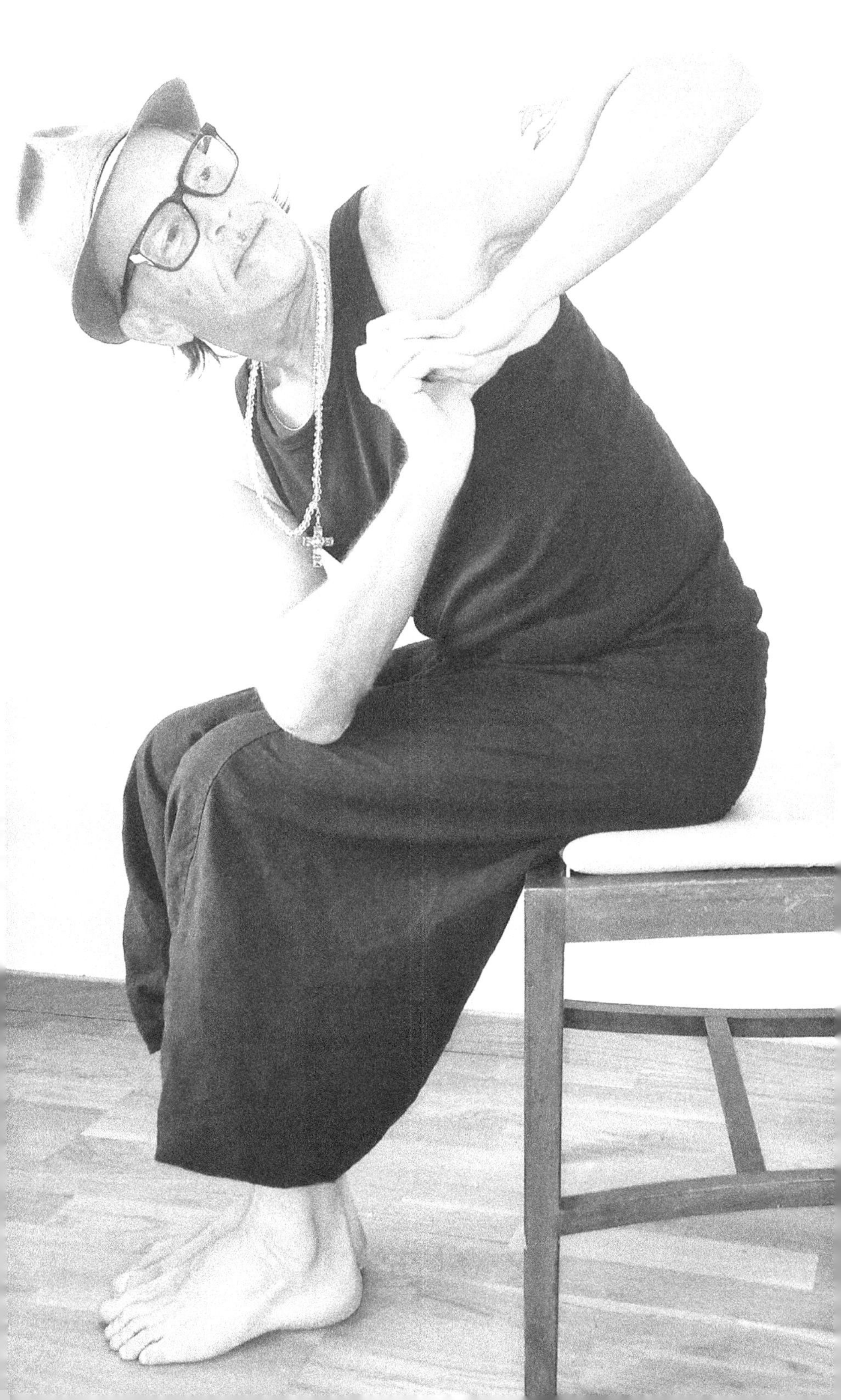

STRENGTH BUILDING FLOW 3

Start by sitting upright on the edge of your chair with your feet flat on the floor and your hands on your thighs. As you inhale, arch your back and push your chest forward for the cat pose.

As you exhale, round your back, pull in your belly, and let your head fall forward. Continue to alternate between these two positions, synchronized with your breath. From the cat pose, gently return to a neutral seated position for a side bend.

Take a deep breath as you lift your left arm overhead with the palm facing inward. Place your right hand beside the chair for stability. Exhale as you bend to the right, creating a "C" shape. You'll feel a nice stretch along your left side. From here, we'll transition directly into an extended side angle or twisted chair.

As you lean to the right, bring down your right forearm to rest on your right thigh and extend your left leg to the side with toes pointing forward. Hold for a few breaths before transitioning to Warrior 1. Keep your legs and left arm still, engage your core as you lift your torso back to the center, rotate your shoulders to the right, and lift your right arm towards the sky. Your arms should be parallel with palms facing each other. Hold for three breaths, and prepare to transition to Warrior 2.

Rotate your shoulders to face the front and lower your arms to the sides until they're at shoulder height. Hold here for three breaths before lowering your arms, returning your left leg to the center, and finishing in mountain pose. Conclude this strength training sequence with the seated pigeon.

Place your left ankle over your right knee. If it feels good, you can stay here. If you want a deeper stretch, gently lean forward from the hips. You should feel a stretch in your right hip and thigh. Repeat the sequence two to three times, then switch sides to complete the sequence two to three times on your left side.

7

CHAIR YOGA
FOR FLEXIBILITY

Yoga is known for promoting increased agility, flexibility, and mobility in the body through a combination of various positions, stretches, and breathing techniques.

Stretches and positions: Yoga encompasses a variety of positions and stretches targeting different muscle groups and joints in the body. By regularly performing these positions, practitioners can gradually increase their agility, mobility, and flexibility. Positions such as forward bends, backward bends, side bends, and twists stretch and loosen the muscles and joints, promoting increased agility and range of motion (Dolgin & Olson, 2017).

Soft tissue work: Many yoga positions involve working with the soft tissues in the body, including muscles, tendons, and connective tissue. By applying gentle tension and pressure to these tissues over extended periods, practitioners can increase blood flow to the area and promote suppleness and elasticity in the tissue. It can help prevent stiffness and promote recovery after exercise or injury (Kong et al., 2016).

Breathwork and relaxation: Yoga also integrates various breathing techniques that can help reduce tension and promote relaxation. Through deep breathing and mindful presence during stretches and positions, practitioners can release muscle tension and enhance their ability to perform stretches comfortably. Muscle relaxation can also promote increased agility by reducing resistance to stretches and movement (Sengupta, 2012).

Injury prevention: Increased agility and mobility can also help prevent injuries by preventing overloading and tension in muscles and joints. By maintaining a smooth and flexible range of motion, practitioners can reduce the risk of muscle strains, ligament injuries, and other injuries during physical activity or daily activities (Bradley et al., 2017).

Mental focus and presence: An essential aspect of yoga is developing conscious presence and mental focus during practice. By being present in the body and aware of one's breathing and body positions, practitioners can enhance their ability to listen to the body's signals and respect their limits during stretches and positions. It can promote a healthy, sustainable practice that supports long-term agility and well-being (Cramer et al., 2016).

In context, yoga offers a holistic approach to increased agility by integrating stretches, soft tissue work, breathwork, injury prevention, and mental focus. By regularly practicing yoga, practitioners can experience various benefits for their mobility and flexibility, translating into improved performance, increased comfort in daily life, and reduced risk of injuries.

REFERENCES

Dolgin, E., & Olson, K. (2017). The science of yoga: The risks and the rewards. National Geographic.

Kong, J., Wilson, G., Park, J., Pereira, K., Walpole, C., Yeates, L., & Janakiraman, B. (2016). The effect of long-duration yoga breath meditation on body awareness and the acquisition of mindfulness: A latent growth curve analysis. Journal of Psychosomatic Research, 89, 21-27.

Sengupta, P. (2012). Health impacts of yoga and pranayama: A state-of-the-art review. International Journal of Preventive Medicine, 3(7), 444-458.

Bradley, K. L., Bushnell, C. A., Davis, G. D., Gorton, B., Slight, S., & Mikalsen, K. H. (2017). Yoga for the prevention and treatment of injury. Journal of Yoga and Physical Therapy, 7(2), 1-7.

Cramer, H., Quinker, D., Schumann, D., Wardle, J., Dobos, G., & Lauche, R. (2016). Adverse effects of yoga: A national cross-sectional survey. BMC complementary and alternative medicine, 16(1), 1-9.

INSTRUCTIONS BEFORE THE YOGA SESSION

Cleanse the nose with a neti pot (a nasal rinsing can with lukewarm water and salt) or nasal spray. Refrain from eating heavy food approximately 2–3 hours before. Preferably, be vegetarian. Do not drink caffeine. All of this calms the mind and gets the blood and prana moving in the body. Sit relaxed with a straight back.

WRIST ROLLS

Wrist rolls are an easy exercise to perform, one that you can do both during and outside of your routine. Keep your hands lightly open, as if holding a handful of eggs you don't want to crush, and rotate your wrists slowly ten times clockwise. When you're done, go in the opposite direction.

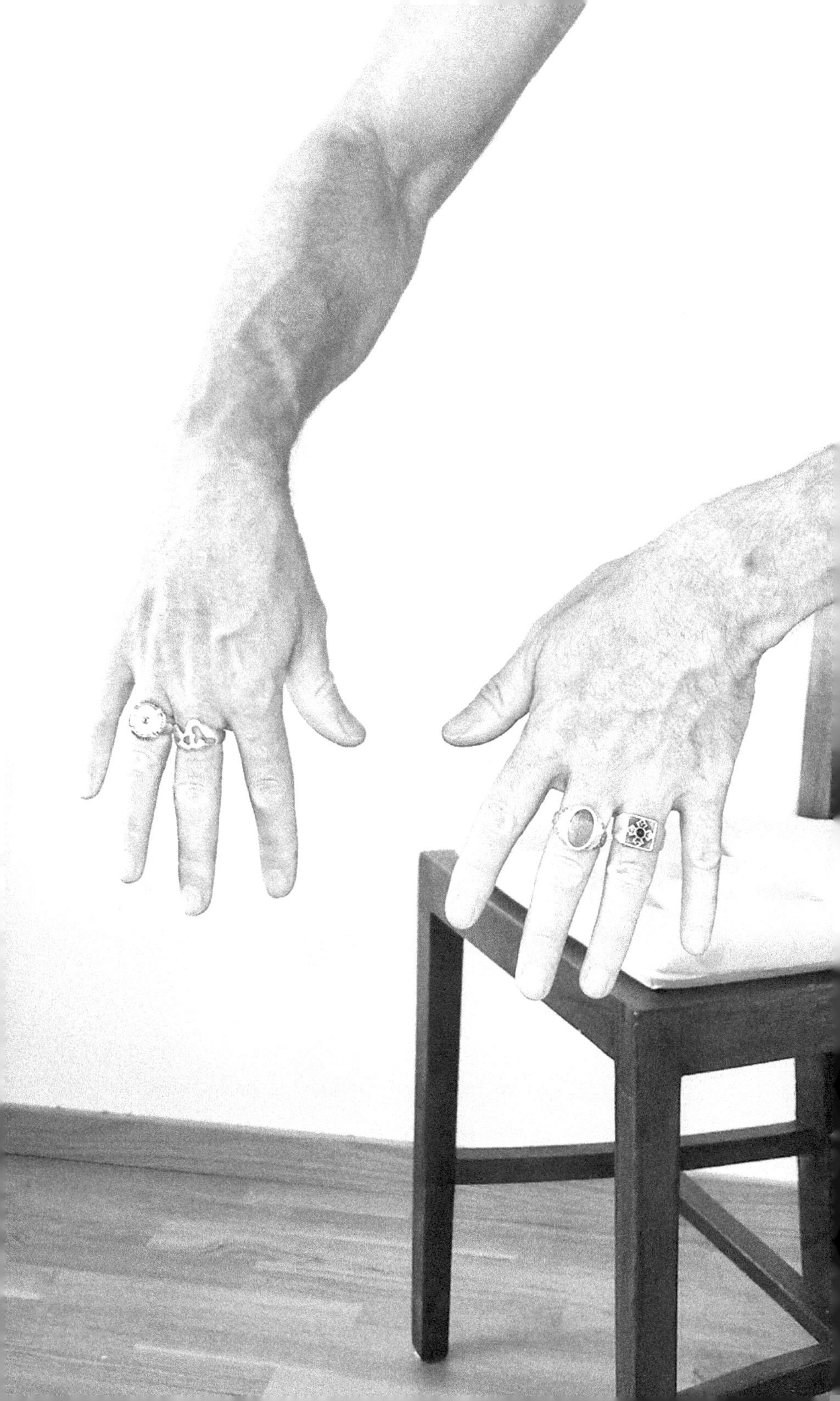

FLOW FOR INCREASED FLEXIBILITY 1

Start by sitting comfortably with your feet flat on the floor and your hands on your thighs or knees with a straight spine. Take a slow, deep breath. On the exhale, lower your chin towards your chest and slowly roll your head clockwise in a large circle, letting it fall backward, then to the right, forward, and left. Repeat this several times in both directions. Be mindful of your movements to ensure it feels good on your neck.

Lift your shoulders towards your ears, then roll them backward, down, and forward in a circular motion. Begin with small rotations and gradually increase to larger ones, then switch direction.

Raise your arms straight in front of you to perform some wrist rolls. Keep your hands lightly open (as if holding a handful of eggs), and then slowly rotate your wrists clockwise – do ten rotations before switching direction.

Next, place your hands on your thighs for cat-cow. As you inhale, arch your back and roll your shoulders down, then lift your chest and gaze upward. As you exhale, round your back, draw your belly in, and let your shoulders and head come forward. Alternate between these two positions several times, syncing your breath with the movement. After your final round of cat, rest with a neutral spine.

Resting your legs straight before you, keeping your feet flexed and active. Place your hands behind your hips with your fingers pointing forward and gently press into your hands to lean your torso forward until you feel a stretch in your calves and hamstrings. Return to the center to repeat the flow.

FLOW FOR INCREASED FLEXIBILITY 2

Begin with shoulder rolls: lift your shoulders towards your ears, then roll them backward, down, and forward in a circular motion. Begin with small rotations and gradually increase to larger ones, then switch direction.

To move into camel pose, roll your shoulders away from your ears and place your palms on your lower back, fingers pointing downward and elbows pointing backward. As you inhale, gently press your hips forward and arch your back, lifting your chest towards the ceiling. You should feel the stretch in your chest. Then, return to a neutral seated position for a forward fold.

Take a deep breath, reach your arms overhead, and lengthen your spine. As you exhale, hinge forward from the hips, allowing your hands to rest on your shins, ankles, or the floor, depending on your flexibility. Let your head hang down for a few breaths, feeling the gentle stretch in your spine. When you're ready, roll your body up to mountain pose. From here, inhale and open your legs into a wide stance, turning your toes outward for a goddess pose.

Lift your arms overhead with palms facing each other and fingers pointing upward. Then, place your hands behind your head and interlock your fingers. Exhale as you lean your torso to the left, pointing your left elbow towards the floor, feeling

*the stretch along your left side. After a few breaths, return
to the center and place your hands on your thighs. Focus on
stretching your right side, then move to the pigeon pose.*

*Place your right ankle over your left knee. Place your hands
in a prayer position and gently lean forward from the hips for
an additional stretch. You should feel a stretch in your right
hip and thigh. After three breaths, lower your right foot to the
floor and return to the center for a spinal twist.*
*Sit up straight and exhale as you twist your torso to the right,
placing your right hand on the back of the chair and your left
hand on your right knee. Look over your right shoulder, hold
for a few breaths, and then inhale to return to the center.*

*Repeat the flow, focusing on your left side during steps four to
six.*

SEATED COW

Sit on your chair with your legs hip-width apart. Extend your right arm over your head and bend the elbow so your hand is along your spine with fingers pointing downward. Use your left hand to bring your right elbow towards the left, allowing your right hand to slide down along your spine. Hold the position for 30 seconds, then switch sides.

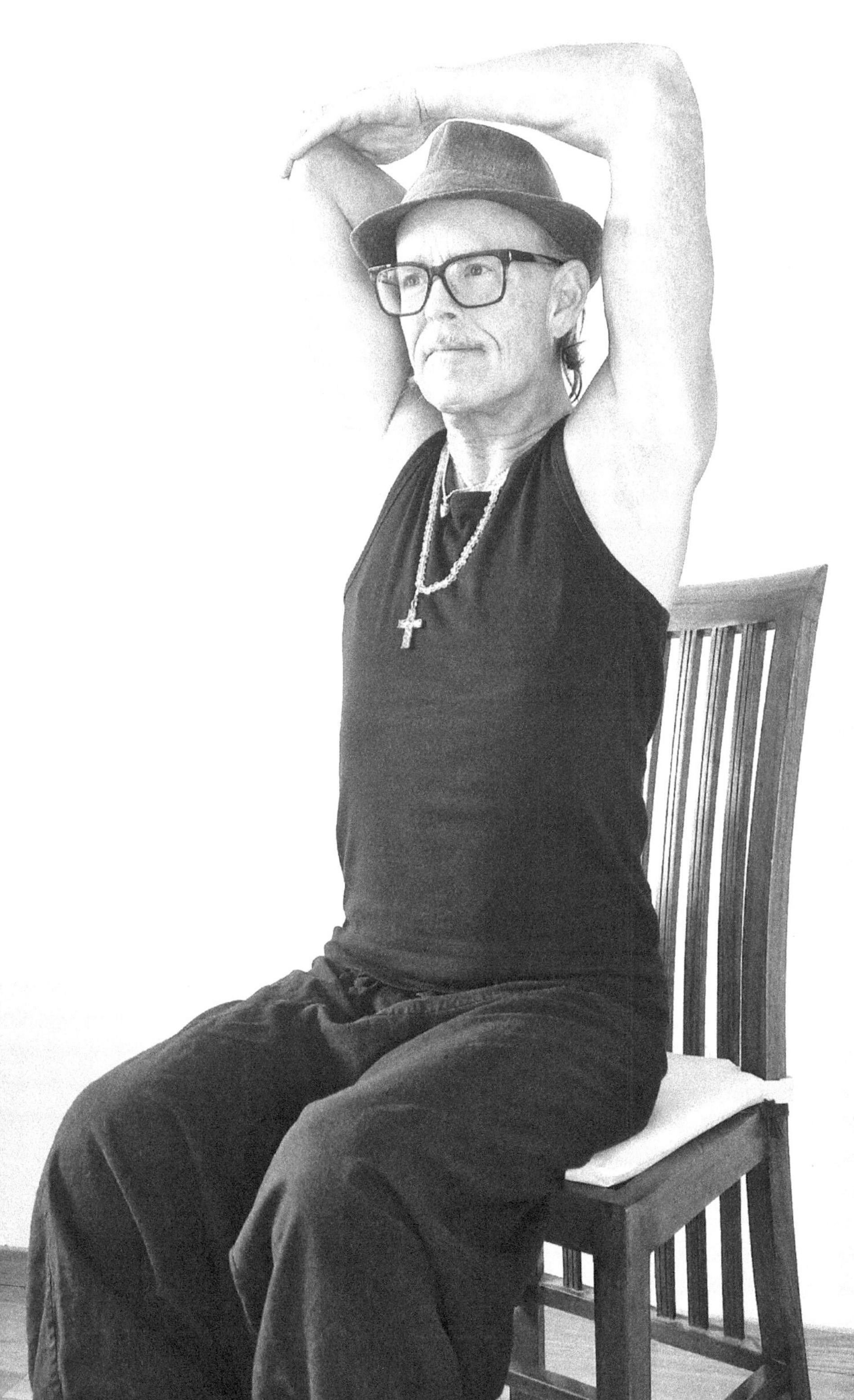

FLOW FOR INCREASED FLEXIBILITY 3

*Raise your arms straight in front of you to perform some wrist
rolls.*

*Keep your hands lightly open (as if holding a handful of eggs),
and then slowly rotate your wrists clockwise—do ten rotations
before switching direction. Slide to the edge of your chair
with a straight spine, feet flat on the floor, and hands on your
thighs. As you inhale, arch your back and push your chest out
for a cat pose.*

*As you exhale, round your back, draw in your belly, and let
your head fall forward. Continue to flow between these two
positions, synchronized with your breath. From the cat pose,
gently return to a neutral seated position for the seated cow
pose.*

*Bend your left arm at the elbow so your fingertips touch your
shoulders. As you extend your right arm overhead, grasp your
left elbow and gently pull to the right. Your left hand will slide
down your spine, giving you a nice stretch in the shoulder,
arm, and back. After three to five breaths, release the arm before switching sides to stretch your right shoulder. After three
to five breaths, inhale deeply as you release your right arm to
lift overhead with the palm facing inward for the side bend.*

Place your left hand on the side of the chair for stability.

Exhale as you lean towards the left, creating a "C" shape. You will feel a nice stretch along your right side; hold for three breaths. From here, keep your left arm lifted as you raise your torso back to a neutral position for an upward plank.

From the mountain pose, move your right leg to the side of your chair as you twist your torso 90 degrees to the right. Place your palms on the chair's seat for support and straighten out your back leg with your toes curled under you. Maintaining a straight spine and engaging your core muscles to find balance. If you're up for the challenge, lift your arms overhead, palms together. After a few breaths, return to the center and repeat the exercise on your opposite side.

8

CHAIR YOGA FOR MORE ENERGY

Yoga, traditionally known for promoting flexibility, relaxation, and mental well-being, has also been shown to improve fitness.

Cardiovascular exercise: Although yoga is not typically considered high-intensity cardiovascular exercise, certain yoga styles and sequences can elevate heart rate and enhance cardiovascular health. Yoga focusing on continuous movements and flows can provide an aerobic training effect and improve fitness by increasing heart rate and enhancing oxygen uptake (Larson-Meyer et al., 2016).

Muscle strength and endurance: Many yoga poses require practitioners to use their body weight as resistance, which can contribute to building muscle strength and endurance over time. Poses such as plank, warrior, and downward dog engage various muscle groups, including core muscles, arms, legs, and back, which can improve muscle tone and endurance (Tran et al., 2016).

Breathing techniques: Yoga integrates various breathing techniques to enhance lung capacity and control. By practicing deep breathing and mindful breathing techniques, practitioners can increase oxygen uptake and improve lung function, which can translate to enhanced endurance and performance during physical activity (Cheema et al., 2015).

Stress management: Stress is a common factor that can negatively impact fitness by increasing cortisol levels and causing muscle tension and fatigue. Yoga effectively reduces stress and promotes relaxation through breathing exercises, meditation, and physical activity. By managing stress, practitioners can improve their endurance and energy levels during exercise and daily activities (Riley et al., 2015).

Holistic well-being: Yoga promotes a holistic approach to health and well-being by integrating physical activity, breathing techniques, and mental relaxation. By enhancing overall well-being and stress management, practitioners may feel more motivated and energetic to engage in regular physical activity and fitness training (Cramer et al., 2018).

In summary, yoga can improve fitness by enhancing cardiovascular exercise, muscle strength and endurance, breath control, stress management, and holistic well-being. By incorporating yoga into their exercise routine, practitioners can experience various benefits for their physical and mental health, contributing to improved fitness and quality of life over time.

REFERENCES

Larson-Meyer, D. E., & Ryschon, T. W. (2016). Yoga Enhances Positive Psychological States in Young Adult Women: A Pilot Study. International Journal of Yoga, 9(2), 161–166.

Tran, M. D., Holly, R. G., Lashbrook, J., & Amsterdam, E. A. (2016). Effects of Hatha Yoga Practice on the Health-Related Aspects of Physical Fitness. Preventive Cardiology, 4(4), 165–170.

Cheema, B. S., Houridis, A., Busch, L., Raschke-Cheema, V., Melville, G. W., & Marshall, P. W. M. (2015). Effect of an office worksite-based yoga program on heart rate variability: outcomes of a randomized controlled trial. BMC Complementary and Alternative Medicine, 15(1), 1–8.

Riley, K. E., Park, C. L., & Wilson, A. (2015). Mindfulness and Affect: A Meta-Analysis of the Effects of Mindfulness Meditation on Affective Outcomes. Journal of Positive Psychology, 10(3), 1–15.

Cramer, H., Ward, L., Steel, A., Lauche, R., Dobos, G., & Zhang, Y. (2018). Prevalence, Patterns, and Predictors of Yoga Use: Results of a U.S. Nationally Representative Survey. American Journal of Preventive Medicine, 55(1), 85–91.

INSTRUCTIONS BEFORE THE YOGA SESSION

Cleanse the nose with a neti pot (a nasal rinsing can with lukewarm water and salt) or nasal spray. Refrain from eating heavy food approximately 2–3 hours before. Preferably, be vegetarian. Do not drink caffeine. All of this calms the mind and gets the blood and prana moving in the body. Sit relaxed with a straight back.

FLOW FOR BETTER FITNESS 1

Sit comfortably on your chair, with your feet firmly planted on the ground as you move through sun salutations. Begin in mountain pose with your knees over your ankles, hip-distance apart. As you inhale deeply, raise your arms overhead and stretch them straight up. Exhale into a prayer position, bringing your hands to your heart center. Keeping your hands in the same position, fold forward by hinging at the hips and rounding your spine. Release your hands and reach them towards your feet. Inhale and roll up, imagining your vertebrae stacking on each other with your head lifting last. Finally, roll your shoulders so they draw away from your ears, and let your hands rest on your thighs as you return to mountain pose.

Continue with the pigeon pose, lifting your right leg and placing your right ankle over your left knee. Bring your hands into a prayer position and gently lean forward, hanging from your hips for an extra stretch. You should feel a stretch in your right hip and glute. After three breaths, lower your right foot to the ground and return to the center for Warrior 2. Move to the right side of your chair, extend your right leg sideways with the knee bent and your right foot flat on the ground. Extend your left leg behind you, toes pointing backward and resting on the ground. Stretch your arms out to the sides at shoulder height, your right arm pointing forward and your left arm pointing backward. Look over your right hand. Hold for a few breaths before transitioning to reverse warrior.

Keep your legs as they are; lower your left hand to rest on the back of your left leg and reach your right arm straight up, stretching your right side. Remember to keep your right knee bent and maintain your balance. From reverse warrior, transition to extended side angle or twisted chair.

Bring both arms to shoulder height as you pass through Warrior 2.

Continue the movement and lower your right forearm to rest on your right thigh while your left arm reaches straight up. Turn your head to the left to look at your fingertips. Hold here for three breaths before returning your torso and arms to the center, passing through Warrior 2 again. As you continue to move, bend your left knee and lift your arms for a chair pose.

As you raise your arms overhead with palms together and

*fingers pointing toward the ceiling, adjust your feet by tur-
ning your toes outward and ensuring your knees remain
directly over your ankles. Then, bend your elbows to 90 degrees, palms facing forward, to create cactus arms. Maintain
your chair pose for the legs, exhale as you twist your body to
the right, gripping the back of your chair with your right arm
and letting your left-hand rest on the outside of your right
thigh. Hold here for a few breaths before slowly twisting for a
forward bend.*

*Move your hands to your inner thighs and inhale to engage
your core muscles. As you exhale, lean forward at your hips
to fold your upper body, ensuring your neck and spine remain
straight and activated. Reach for the floor, or let your hands
rest on your knees. Remember to listen to your body and only
fold forward as far as feels good. Hang here for a few breaths,
releasing tension in your lower back and hips. Slowly lift your
torso back to the chair pose.*

*Repeat this flow two or four times, focusing on both the left
and right sides.*

MOUNTAIN WITH SQUAT

Start by sitting on your chair with your hands hanging at your sides. Extend your arms at shoulder height as you lift your buttocks from the chair to a standing position. Slowly lower back down to your chair. Stand up again and repeat steps two through four.

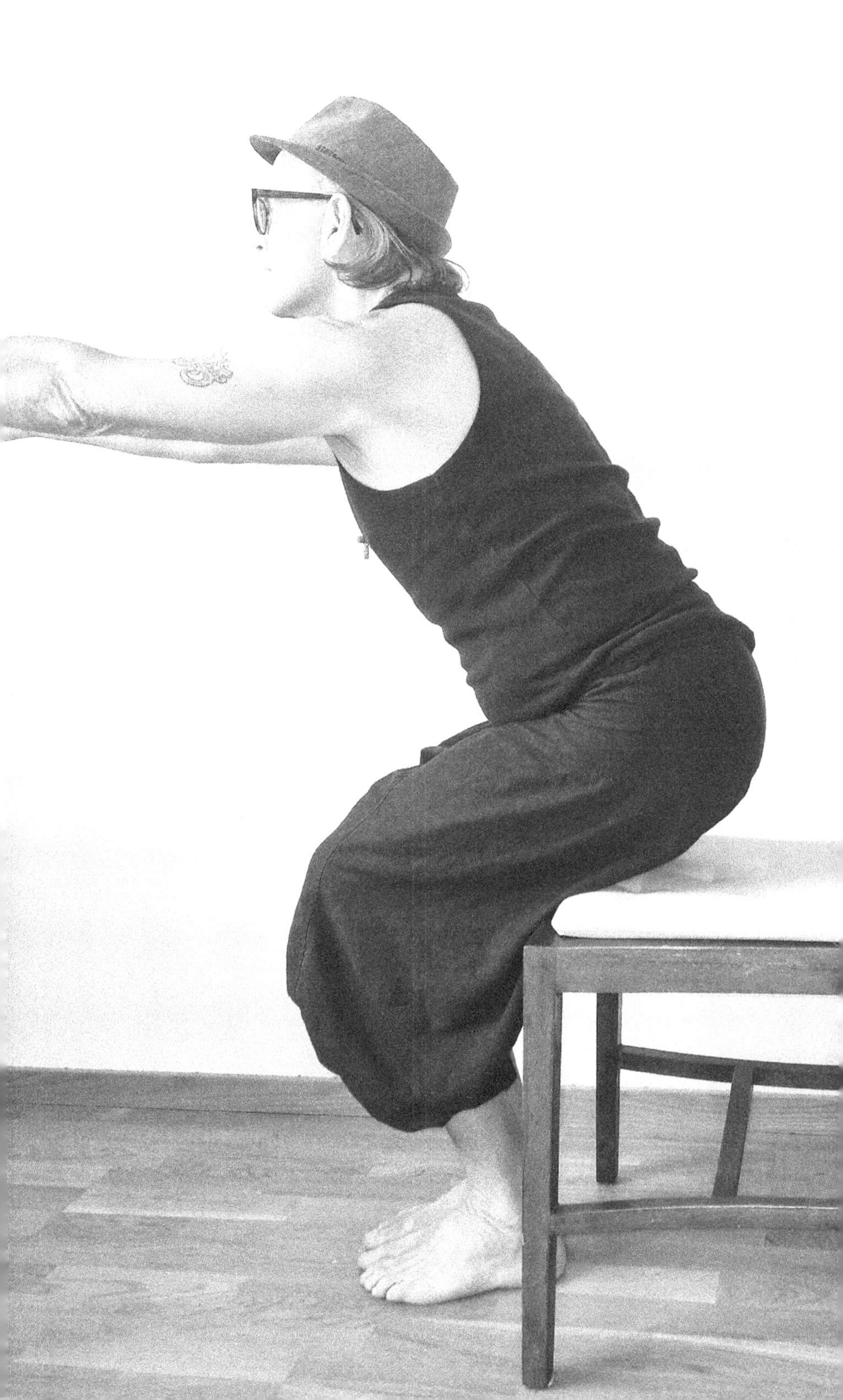

FLOW FOR BETTER FITNESS 2

Start with the sun salutation. Begin in a mountain pose with your knees directly above your ankles, a hip distance apart. As you inhale deeply, raise your arms overhead and stretch them straight up. Exhale into a prayer position as you bring your hands to your heart center. Keeping your hands in the same position, fold forward by hinging at the hips and rounding your spine. Release your hands and reach them towards your feet. Inhale and roll up, imagining your vertebrae stacking on each other with your head lifting last. Finally, roll your shoulders so they draw away from your ears, and let your hands rest on your thighs as you return to mountain pose to prepare for a spinal twist.

Bring your feet together and engage your inner thigh muscles by squeezing your knees as you bring your hands to a prayer position in the middle of your chest. Twist your torso to the right so that your right elbow points towards the ceiling and your left elbow rests outside your right knee. Ensure you do not release your shoulders but roll them back to create a straight line from elbow to elbow. Hold for three breaths before returning to the center. After three breaths, return to the center and prepare to work with the legs.

Extend your arms forward at shoulder height as you lift your buttocks from the chair, just enough to engage your leg muscles but not enough to stand completely. Lower back onto your chair, and then stand up again to repeat the process. After your final squat, sit back on your chair to prepare for a more significant movement.

Inhale deeply, and as you exhale, simultaneously push up through your feet and lift your arms to shoulder height to stand up. Once standing, lower your arms back down to your sides. Inhale as you sit down, and your arms repeat the process. Repeat this position a few times to synchronize your movement with your breath.

Now, let's engage our core with the boat pose. With the desired variation, lean back slightly, lift one or both legs, and cross your fingers behind the knee. Activate your core as you hold the position and avoid rounding your back. If you're ready for an extra challenge, unlock your fingers and lift your arms. Hold three breaths before lowering one or both legs and returning to the mountain pose. Repeat steps one through five.

Enter camel pose. Place your palms on your lower back, fingers pointing downwards and elbows pointing backward. As you inhale, gently press your hips forward and arch your back, lifting your chest towards the ceiling. If you feel balanced, lean back to gaze up at the ceiling. You should feel the stretch in your chest and core. Then, return to a neutral seated position to conclude the flow in the child's pose.

Open your legs slightly wider than hip-width apart. Inhale to lengthen your spine, then exhale and bend forward, allowing your arms to rest on a chair before you or letting your finger-tips reach the floor.

FLOW FOR BETTER FITNESS 3

Begin in a mountain pose by sitting tall on the edge of your chair, with your feet flat on the floor and hip-distance apart. Inhale and stretch your arms overhead, bringing your palms together. Interlace your fingers while keeping your index and thumbs out to point towards the ceiling. Exhale and roll your shoulders away from your ears. Hold here for five breaths before releasing your arms and slowly lowering them to the sides until they reach the sides of your chair.

Place your palms on the seat just behind your buttocks with your knuckles facing forward to prepare for an upward plank.

Extend both legs diagonally in front of you with your toes flexed towards the ceiling. Press into your hands and feet and engage your core as you lift your buttocks off the chair to create a straight line with your body. Hold for two to three breaths before slowly lowering back to your chair and preparing for mountain pose with squat.

From the mountain pose, inhale deeply, and as you exhale, push up through your feet and lift your arms to shoulder height to stand up. Once standing, lower your arms back down to your sides. Inhale as you sit down, and your arms repeat the process. Complete this position a few times, and on your final repetition, remain standing.

Twist your body to face the seat of your chair. Take one or two steps back to be comfortable from the chair and perform an upward plank. Place your left foot on the chair, press into both feet for support, and place your hands on your hips. Ensure to position the chair against a wall to avoid unwanted movement. You can also turn the chair so the backrest is sideways and hold onto it for additional support. Hold the stretch for five breaths before switching sides. Face the chair, place your hands on the seat, and step back until your body is straight from head to heel. Engage your core and hold the plank for a few breaths.

To transition from plank to standing mountain pose, engage your core, lift your hips, and push them back. Ensure you are solid and stable in your shoulders and arms. Hold a few breaths before lowering your knees to the floor to return to a seated position.

Continue with the forward fold. Sit comfortably on your chair and inhale as you reach up, then exhale and bend forward, releasing tension in your neck and shoulders. Let your arms rest on the chair or release them to the floor. Hold for a few breaths before slowly rolling up to finish.

Sit comfortably on your chair, close your eyes, and take a few deep breaths to ground yourself. Notice how your body feels now compared to when you started this flow. Imagine rele-

asing tensions and worries with each exhale and allowing calmness and peace to fill you with each inhale.

Stay here for as long as it feels peaceful.

9

CHAIR YOGA
FOR WEIGHT LOSS

Yoga may be one of many activities that come to mind when discussing weight loss. Still, research has shown that regular yoga can be an effective complementary method for achieving and maintaining a healthy weight.

Physical activity: Although some yoga styles are less intense than other forms of exercise, yoga still involves physical activity that can contribute to calorie burning and thus lead to weight loss. Dynamic yoga styles like Vinyasa and Ashtanga can increase heart rate and burn calories, similar to other cardiovascular exercises (Kristal et al., 2005).

Muscle building: Yoga often requires bearing one's body weight in various positions, thereby strength training different muscle groups. By increasing muscle mass, yoga can boost overall metabolism and calorie burning, even at rest (Hunter et al., 2013).

Stress reduction: Stress can lead to weight gain by increasing cortisol production, a hormone that can increase appetite and lead to overeating. Yoga effectively reduces stress and promotes relaxation, which can help reduce appetite and prevent overeating related to emotional stress (Daubenmier et al., 2016).

Mindful eating: A central principle in yoga is awareness, including when it comes to food. By practicing mindful eating, yoga practitioners can learn to listen to their body's hunger signals and eat more healthily, leading to better weight management (Timmerman & Brown, 2012).

Improvement in sleep: Inadequate sleep has been linked to weight gain and difficulties in losing weight. Yoga can improve sleep by promoting relaxation and reducing sleep disturbances, supporting weight loss and maintenance (Halpern et al., 2014).

Metabolic health: Research has shown that yoga can improve metabolic markers such as blood sugar levels, insulin sensitivity, and lipid profile, which can promote weight loss and reduce the risk of metabolic diseases like diabetes and cardiovascular disease (Innes & Vincent, 2007).

Regular yoga can be integral to healthy weight management by increasing physical activity, promoting muscle building and metabolism, reducing stress, and promoting mindful eating and sound sleep. Combining yoga with a balanced diet and other forms of exercise can be an effective strategy for achieving and maintaining a healthy weight over time.

REFERENCES

Kristal, A. R., Littman, A. J., Benitez, D., & White, E. (2005). Yoga practice is associated with attenuated weight gain in healthy, middle-aged men and women. Alternative Therapies in Health and Medicine, 11(4), 28–33.

Hunter, S. D., Dhindsa, M. S., & Cunningham, E. (2013). Tarahumara Medicine: Ethnobotany and Healing among the Rarámuri of Mexico. University of Oklahoma Press.

Daubenmier, J., Kristeller, J., Hecht, F. M., Maninger, N., Kuwata, M., Jhaveri, K., … Epel, E. (2016). Mindfulness Intervention for Stress Eating to Reduce Cortisol and Abdominal Fat among Overweight and Obese Women: An Exploratory Randomized Controlled Study. Journal of Obesity, 2011, 1–13.

Timmerman, G. M., & Brown, A. (2012). The Effect of a Mindful Restaurant Eating Intervention on Weight Management in Women. Journal of Nutrition Education and Behavior, 44(1), 22–28.

Halpern, J., Cohen, M., Kennedy, G., Reece, J., & Cahan, C. (2014). Yoga for improving sleep quality and quality of life for older adults. Alternative Therapies in Health and Medicine, 20(3), 37–46.

Innes, K. E., & Vincent, H. K. (2007). The influence of yoga-based programs on risk profiles in adults with type 2 diabetes mellitus: A systematic review. Evidence-Based Complementary and Alternative Medicine, 4(4), 469–486.

INSTRUCTIONS BEFORE THE YOGA SESSION

Cleanse the nose with a neti pot (a nasal rinsing can with lukewarm water and salt) or nasal spray. Refrain from eating heavy food approximately 2–3 hours before. Preferably, be vegetarian. Do not drink caffeine. All of this calms the mind and gets the blood and prana moving in the body. Sit relaxed with a straight back.

STANDING WIND RELIEVING POSE

The standing wind–relieving pose is a standing variation of the seated one. Pulling your leg towards your chest should cause you to get a deeper stretch in your glute muscles.

Stand with your back to your chair on the left side. Place your left hand on the backrest for support with your right hand on your hip. Lift your right leg as high as it can go. You can grasp your knee with your right hand to pull it closer to your chest. Ensure that your spine remains straight. Hold the position for a few moments, then lower it again. Perform ten repetitions before switching sides.

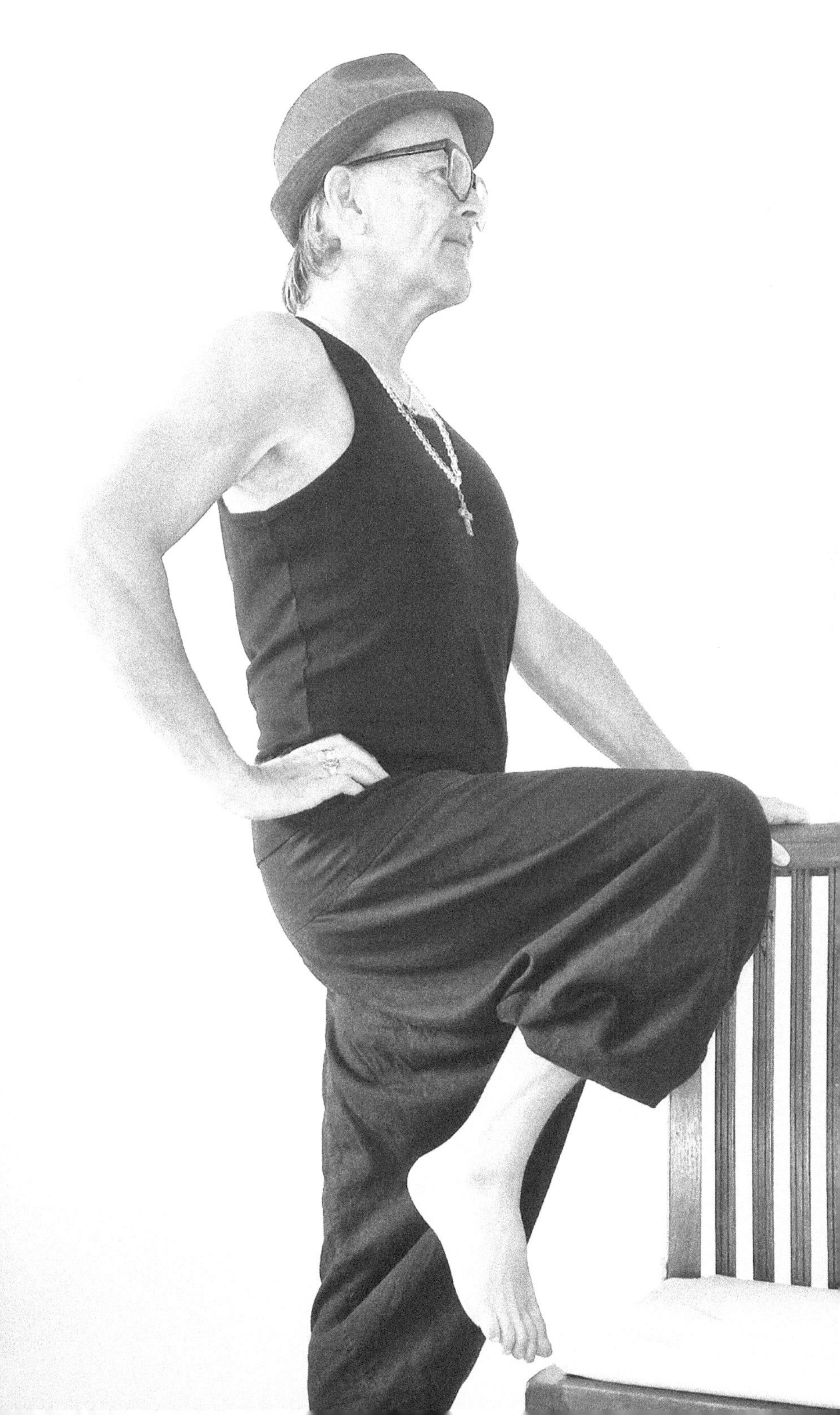

WEIGHT LOSS FLOW 1

Stand up and place your left hand on the backrest for support, with your right hand on your hip. Lift your right leg as high as it can go. You can grab your knee with your right hand to pull it closer to your chest. Ensure that your spine remains straight. Hold for a few moments and then lower it again. Do ten repetitions before switching sides.

Continue with the standing mountain pose. Stand a short distance from the front of the chair, bend your torso towards the chair's seat, and adjust your feet until your body forms an excellent "V" shape, with your hips at the highest point. Press your palms against the chair, draw in your abdomen, and push your hips backward. Your head should be in line with your arms. Hold here for a couple of breaths.

We'll first pass through the upward plank to transition to the cobra. Lean forward at the hips until your body is straight from head to heel. Activate your core for a few breaths. After your last exhale, exhale and lift your chest until you have a slight arch in your back. Hold for two to three breaths.

Walk your feet toward the front of the chair until you reach a standing position.

Move into a triangle pose, stepping forward with your right leg just behind the chair and your left leg about two to th–

ree steps behind, toes pointing forward. Shift your left hip back and lower your right hand until it reaches the chair seat while stretching your left arm toward the ceiling. Turn your head left to look up at your fingertips. It should create a nice straight line from your left hand to your right. Remember to keep both legs straight and your chest open as you hold for three breaths. Go to the side of your chair so the backrest is on your left side for standing wind relieving.

Place your left hand on the backrest and your right hand on your hip. Ensure your spine remains straight, and lift your right leg as high as possible. You can use your right hand to pull your leg closer to your chest if you want. Hold this position briefly before lowering your leg and preparing for an upward plank.

Turn the chair so that your left hand is on the backrest and your right foot is on the seat. Adjust your feet until you feel comfortable making a high plank from the chair. Place your right leg on the chair, press down on both feet for support, and place your hands on your hips. Hold the stretch for five breaths before setting your foot back on the floor. Repeat all steps, focusing on your left side for the standing wind-relieving position and the high plank.

WEIGHT LOSS FLOW 2

Begin in mountain pose with hands on knees. On an inhale, lift your arms overhead with palms facing each other and fingers pointing towards the ceiling. Keep your spine straight as you exhale, and press your weight through your heels to partially stand up from your chair until your legs are about 45 degrees. Hold about three to five breaths before shifting to sit on the chair again, preparing for the boat pose.

With the boat pose in mind, slide to the front of the chair, lean back slightly, lift one or both legs, and clasp your fingers behind your knee. Activate your core as you hold the position and avoid rounding your back. If you're ready for an extra challenge, unlock your fingers and lift your arms. Hold for three breaths before lowering one or both legs and returning to mountain pose for Warrior 2.

Move to the right side of your chair, extend your right leg sideways with the knee bent and your right foot flat on the floor. Extend your left leg behind you, toes pointing backward and resting on the floor. Stretch your arms sideways at shoul-der height, your right arm pointing forward and your left arm pointing backward, looking over your proper fingertips. Hold for a few breaths before transitioning to reverse warrior.

Keep your legs as they are. Lower your left hand to rest on the back of your left leg, and stretch your right arm up towards the ceiling, creating a nice stretch on your right side. Remember to keep the right knee bent and maintain your balance. While holding the reverse warrior position, let's transition to an extended side angle or twisted chair.

Bring both arms to shoulder height as you pass back through Warrior 2. Continue the movement and lower your right forearm to rest on your right thigh while your left arm points towards the sky. Turn your head to the left to look at your fingertips. Hold here for three breaths before repeating the routine.

WEIGHT LOSS FLOW 3

Start by ensuring that your chair is stable and doesn't slide. Begin with triangle pose.

Stand in front of your chair with feet hip-width apart. Step your right leg forward so it's just behind the chair, and your left leg is behind, about two to three steps, with toes pointing forward. Shift your left hip back and lower your right hand until it reaches the chair seat while stretching your left arm toward the ceiling. Turn your head left to look up at your fingertips. It should create a nice straight line from your left hand to your right. Remember to keep both legs straight and your chest open as you hold for three breaths. Go into standing mountain pose.

Rotate your shoulders to the right until they face the chair's seat. Place your hands on the seat shoulder-width apart before adjusting your feet to form the iconic "V" shape. Press your palms against the chair, draw in your abdomen, and shift your hips backward. Your head should be in line with your arms. Hold here for a few breaths before moving your feet back towards the chair for Warrior 1.

Sit on the edge of your chair, tall with feet flat on the floor. Rotate to the right so your right leg is bent over the side of the chair and your right foot is flat on the floor. Extend your left leg behind you, toes pointing backward and resting on the floor. Sweep your arms up towards the sky and take a moment to find your balance. While keeping your leg positions, only rotate your upper body to the left, lowering your arms to shoulder height, with your right arm pointing forward and your left arm pointing backward. Keep both legs as they are, lower your left arm to rest on the back of your left leg, and stretch your right arm towards the ceiling, creating a nice stretch on your right side. Remember to keep the right knee bent and maintain your balance.

After three breaths, slowly lift your torso and bring your body back to the center. Then, return to mountain pose but with your feet together for a twisted chair.

*Squeeze your knees to activate your inner thigh muscles as you bring your hands to a prayer position in the middle of your chest. As you bend at your hips, twist your torso to the right so that your right elbow points towards the ceiling and your left elbow rests outside your right knee. Roll back your shoulders to create a straight line from elbow to elbow. Hold for five breaths before twisting back to the center.
Repeat the flow, focusing on the left side.*

10

RELAXATION & MEDITATION

Meditation has long been known for its positive effects on health and well-being, and research has increasingly confirmed its many benefits. By reducing stress and promoting inner calm, meditation can be a powerful resource for improving physical and mental health.

A study published in the journal "JAMA Internal Medicine" found that mindfulness meditation reduced levels of the stress hormone cortisol in participants, resulting in improved feelings of well-being and reduced experience of stress.

Research has also shown that meditation can positively affect the brain and cognitive functions. A meta-analysis published in the journal "Neuroscience & Biobehavioral Reviews" found that meditation can increase gray matter volume in the brain, linked to improved cognitive function and reduced age-related decline in brain tissue.

Meditation has also been shown to have beneficial effects on the physical level. A review article published in the journal

Annals of the New York Academy of Sciences summarized research showing that meditation can lower blood pressure, reduce inflammation, and improve immune system function.

In addition to its physical and mental health benefits, meditation can also promote emotional balance and increase emotional intelligence. A study published in the journal Psychological Science found that regular meditation increased participants' ability to manage negative emotions and emotional stability.

In summary, research has clearly shown that meditation can positively affect health and well-being. By reducing stress, improving cognitive functions, promoting emotional balance, and supporting physical health, meditation can be a powerful resource for promoting an overall healthy lifestyle and increasing quality of life.

REFERENCES

Rosenkranz, M. A., Davidson, R. J., Maccoon, D. G., Sheridan, J. F., Kalin, N. H., & Lutz, A. (2013). A comparison of mindfulness-based stress reduction and an active control in modulation of neurogenic inflammation. Brain, Behavior, and Immunity, 27(1), 174-184.

Fox, K. C., Nijeboer, S., Dixon, M. L., Floman, J. L., Ellamil, M., Rumak, S. P., ... & Christoff, K. (2014). Is meditation associated with altered brain structure? A systematic review and meta-analysis of morphometric neuroimaging in meditation practitioners. Neuroscience & Biobehavioral Reviews, 43, 48-73.

Pascoe, M. C., Thompson, D. R., Jenkins, Z. M., & Ski, C. F. (2017). Mindfulness mediates the physiological markers of stress: Systematic review and meta-analysis. Journal of Psychiatric Research, 95, 156-178.

Desbordes, G., Negi, L. T., Pace, T. W., Wallace, B. A., Raison, C. L., & Schwartz, E. L. (2012). Effects of mindful-attention and compassion meditation training on amygdala response to emotional stimuli in an ordinary, non-meditative state. Frontiers in Human Neuroscience, 6, 292.

YOGA NIDRA

Yogic deep relaxation/meditation.

Yoga Nidra, also known as yogic sleep, is a unique medita-tion practice that is deeply powerful and healing for the body, mind, and soul. It has its roots in the oldest Indian and tantric scriptures. It was originally developed from the tantric nyasa techniques, which were used to incorporate and vitalize the body and mind with universal energy. Specific mantras are placed on various parts of the body to activate energy centers and release blockages along the subtle energy channel known as nadis and energy centers known as chakras.

According to tantric traditions, the foundation of nyasa tech-niques lies in achieving a deeper awareness of the body and energy flow and attaining a profound spiritual understanding and experience. By focusing the mind on different body parts and visualizing specific mantras or sounds, the practitioner can create a strong connection between body, mind, and spirit and achieve a sense of inner balance and harmony.

Yoga Nidra, which evolved from these nyasa techniques, is a form of guided meditation and relaxation where practitioners are guided through a series of steps to achieve deep relaxation and awareness. During a typical Yoga Nidra session, participants are led through a systematic relaxation exercise that includes body awareness, breathing exercises, visualizations, and affirmations to promote deep relaxation and inner stillness.

The benefits of Yoga Nidra include reduced stress and anxiety, improved sleep quality, increased body awareness and relaxation, and promoting inner peace and well-being. Through regular practice of Yoga Nidra, the practitioner can experience a sense of deep inner calm and peace as well as increased clarity and concentration.

The original nyasa techniques and their philosophy and practice can be found in several classic tantric texts, including Tantrasara, Vijnanabhairava Tantra, and Shiva Svarodaya. These texts offer insights and guidance on practicing nyasa to enhance the mind and experience more profound awareness and spirituality. Exploring these texts with the help of authorized teachers and guides can be a way to understand and appreciate the rich tradition of Nyasa and its role in the development of Yoga Nidra and other meditation techniques.

Yoga Nidra offers comprehensive benefits but is one of the most straightforward yoga practices. All you need to do is put on your most comfortable clothes, find a quiet space, sit on a comfy chair, or lie on your back and listen to the meditation (the link to YouTube can be found on page 5 of the book). If you prefer to practice sitting, you can also practice Yoga Nidra with open eyes, focusing your gaze on the center of the kaleidoscope.

INSTRUCTIONS

Sitting comfortably on a chair or lying on a mat.

Instructions for sitting: Cleanse the nose with a neti pot or nasal spray. Avoid eating heavy meals about 2-3 hours before. Preferably vegetarian. Avoid drinking caffeine. All of this calms the mind and regulates the blood and prana in the body. Sit relaxed with a straight back. Close your eyes or gently squint at the centering in the middle of the kaleidoscope. You will notice that your entire chakra system activates instantly. If you feel tired, close your eyes and continue listening.

Instructions for lying down: Cleanse the nose with a neti pot or nasal spray. Avoid eating heavy meals about 2-3 hours before. Preferably vegetarian. Avoid drinking caffeine. All of this calms the mind and regulates the blood and prana in the body. Please wear your most comfortable clothes, find a quiet space, lie on your back, and play the sleep meditation (available on my YouTube). Listen attentively. Do not fall asleep. If you feel drowsy, raise one forearm. If it falls, you will be awakened.

Your sankalpa (your decision and desire) should never be revealed to anyone. Doing so diminishes its power.

INTRODUCTION (*Sitting*)

Prepare yourself for yoga nidra. Sit down and adjust your clothes so you are comfortable and don't need to move anymore. Now, focus on the body. Become aware of the body's stillness. You sit completely still as if the body were made of stone. Aware of the body – body awareness. Listen to all the sounds around you. All sounds simultaneously, effortlessly. Tell yourself … I am awake and will practice yoga nidra; I will not fall asleep.

Now it's time to make your decision—your sankalpa. Be positive, clear, and distinct. Say it silently to yourself three times. It will settle deep into your subconscious and be bound to manifest.

Repeat the body parts after me mentally and fill them with your awareness…

Move to your right hand…
Thumb on your right side, index finger, middle finger, ring finger, little finger, hand, arm, shoulder, armpit, chest, abdomen, thigh, knee, shin, foot, big toe, second toe, third toe, fourth toe, and little toe, experience your entire right side…

Take your awareness to your left side…
experience your left thumb, index finger, etc…

Experience the back of your head, neck, shoulders, spine, entire back... buttocks, thighs, back of the knee, calves, and feet... experience your entire back...

Experience the top of the head, forehead, nose, tip of the nose, lips, chin, chin tip, throat, collarbone, chest, arms, navel, inside the navel, genitals, thighs, knees, shins, feet, toes... Experience the entire right arm, entire left arm, entire right leg, left leg, torso, head... the whole body...

Now focus on the breath...
experience it, do not control it... move to the left nostril, feel how you inhale and how it exits through the right nostril..., and feel the temperature difference at the upper lip... On 1, inhale through the left nostril; on 1, exhale through the right; on 2, inhale through the right; and on 2, exhale through the left... on 5, 10, 15, etc., inhale through both nostrils and exhale through both. Count carefully; if you make a mistake, start over from 1... (alternate nostril breathing)...

See the following objects in front of you, touch them, smell them...
a desert, pyramid, temple, a Buddha statue, a rose, waves far out to sea, flame, sunrise, birds flying, clouds... yin and yang, Shiva, a triangle with the tip pointing downwards, a triangle with the tip pointing upwards, lying on top of each other to form a six-pointed star, a circle, a square, experience happi-

ness, a golden egg, a pulsating white light at the center of the eyebrows... a thousand-petaled lotus flower at the top of your head...

237

Now it's time to repeat your decision, your sankalpa—clear and distinct—three times. Chant Hari Om Tat Sat three times, and then yoga nidra is over for this time.

We can now open our eyes and start moving our bodies...

AJAPA JAPA

Classic yogic meditation with the mantra So-Ham.

Ajapa Japa is a form of meditation rooted in the Vedic tradi-tion and is a powerful technique for calming the mind and deepening awareness. "Ajapa" means "that which happens spontaneously by itself," and "Japa" refers to the repeti-tion of a mantra or sacred sound. In Ajapa Japa meditation, breathing techniques are integrated with the repetition of a mantra to create a deep and immersive meditation practice.

Ajapa Japa, which has its roots in the ancient yogic scriptu-res, has been practiced by yogis and monks for centuries to achieve spiritual realization and inner peace. The technique focuses on harmonizing the breath with the repetition of a mantra, helping practitioners attain a deeper level of conscio-usness and stillness of mind.

In Ajapa Japa meditation, the practitioner coordinates inha-lation and exhalation by repeating a mantra, usually "So-

Ham," which means "I am that" in Sanskrit. "So" is repeated in mind during inhalation and exhalation, and "Ham" is repeated. By harmonizing the breath with the mantra, a meditative rhythm is created that helps to calm the mind and opens doors to deep inner stillness and awareness.

There are many benefits to Ajapa Japa meditation, including both physical and mental benefits. By integrating breathing techniques with mantra repetition, practitioners can experience the following benefits:

Reduced stress and anxiety: By deepening awareness and calming the mind, Ajapa Japa meditation can reduce stress levels and promote inner peace and tranquility.

Improved concentration: The repetitive nature of the mantra helps to focus the mind and enhance concentration, which can be beneficial both in meditation and daily life.

Increased awareness: By deepening awareness and presence in the present moment, Ajapa Japa meditation can raise awareness of one's inner state and promote self-awareness and personal growth.

Enhanced mental control: By practicing following the breath and repeating the mantra, practitioners can develop increased cognitive control and self-regulation, which can be beneficial for managing emotional reactions and impulsivity.

Improved sleep quality: Many people find that regular meditation, including Ajapa Japa, can enhance sleep quality by reducing stress and promoting relaxation.

INSTRUCTIONS

Sitting comfortably on a chair or lying on a mat. Put on your most comfortable clothes, find a quiet space, sit on a comfy chair, or lie on your back and listen to the meditation (the link to YouTube is on page 5). If you prefer to practice sitting, you can also practice Ajapa Japa with your eyes open, focusing on the center of the kaleidoscope.

Instructions for sitting: Cleanse your nose with a neti pot (nasal rinsing can with lukewarm water and salt) or nasal spray. Avoid eating heavy meals about 2-3 hours before. Preferably vegetarian. Avoid caffeine. All of this calms the mind and facilitates blood and prana flow in the body. Sit relaxed with a straight back. Close your eyes or gently squint at the centering in the middle of the kaleidoscope. You will notice that your entire chakra system activates immediately. If you feel tired, close your eyes and continue listening.

Instructions for lying down: Cleanse your nose with a neti pot (nasal rinsing can with lukewarm water and salt) or nasal spray. Avoid eating heavy meals about 2-3 hours before. Preferably vegetarian. Avoid caffeine. All of this calms the mind and facilitates blood and prana flow in the body. Please wear your most comfortable clothes, find a quiet space, lie on your back, and listen to the meditation (available on my YouTube channel). Listen attentively. Do not fall asleep. If you feel drowsy, raise one forearm. If it falls, you will wake up.

INTRODUCTION

Sit in a comfortable meditation posture and be aware of your body. Take a moment to adjust your position, feel if your legs and feet are correctly placed, and change your position, if necessary, now before the meditation begins. Choose the position carefully; you should be able to sit in it as comfortably as possible without needing to move...

Take a deep breath and stretch your entire spine toward the ceiling. On exhalation, relax, but maintain the stretch in the back. Relax the facial muscles, forehead, eyelids, cheeks, lips, tongue, and lower jaw. Relax the arms, letting the hands rest on the knees or in the lap completely relaxed. Relax the buttocks, legs, and feet.

STEP 1. EXPERIENCE OF BREATHING

Experience the movement in the abdomen and chest... the abdomen expanding on inhalation... the abdomen contracting on exhalation... Feel the airflow through both nostrils... calm, steady rhythm... Be aware of the sound of breathing... natural rhythm...

STEP 2. ACTIVATE THE YOGIC BREATH

Imagine the breath's movement in a passage between the navel and the throat: Breathe in from the navel to the throat, hold the breath at the throat, say Vishuddhi three times, then breathe down to the navel, hold the breath out, say Manipura three times, then breathe up to the throat, etc.

STEP 3. UJJAYI PRANAYAMA

Activate ujjayi pranayama and kechari mudra. Breathe with a hissing sound from the throat (ujjayi pranayama, children often say it sounds like Darth Vader in Star Wars). Then, continue the tongue to the palate (kechari mudra).

STEP 4. MANTRA SO-HAM

Be fully aware of the mantra in coordination with the breath... So ... o with inhalation... Ha ... am with exhalation.

EXPANSION OF AWARENESS

If thoughts or feelings spontaneously arise, be aware of them, but let them disappear like small clouds...

Remind yourself of this several times during ongoing meditation. Strive to develop an active and conscious attitude.

ENDING

Say Hari Om Tat Sat silently to yourself three times.

You can return to your natural breathing, cease the experience of the passage and our two chakras, stop the mantra, gently open your eyes, and start moving your body...

11

THE SPIRITUAL ASPECT

THE SPIRITUAL ASPECT

When you've been practicing yoga for a while, things start to happen in your consciousness. Slowly, your awareness begins to expand. It means stepping out of your head and your usual thought patterns to suddenly become a witness. Gradually, you develop an attitude of witnessing towards yourself, your fellow human beings, and the environment at large. Consciousness is no longer confined to form; it becomes formless and can expand. Tanoti and Tayatri. Tantra. Expansion and liberation.

During yoga, the mind quiets down, and suddenly, you become aware of all the emotions and thoughts surfacing. You gain insight into destructive thought patterns and habits you tend to get stuck in, what really matters for your positive development, and where true happiness actually comes from. Suddenly, you realize that joy always exists within you, but it's hidden when you're not balanced and not what is called Sattvik in Sanskrit.

That happiness is accurate, not just a pleasurable sensation like winning a competition. Because happiness linked to achievement isn't sustainable in the long run. No, it needs to be chased, constantly achieved, and experienced, like when people who seemingly have everything still feel lost and empty.

According to Buddhist tradition, Siddhartha Gautama, later known as Buddha, left his life as a prince and sought enlightenment by wandering in the forests of India. During his quest for insight, he encountered many yogis and ascetics and explored various forms of meditation and asceticism.

During his quest, Buddha devoted much time to training with yogic monks and masters. Their teachings and methods contributed to Buddha's understanding of the body and mind and the development of the meditation practice that would later become known as the core of Buddhism.

The yogic monks' training focused on many principles that Buddha would later teach, including meditation, mindfulness, and insight into the true nature of things. They also taught techniques to control the mind and achieve inner peace and balance.

Through his experiences with the yogic monks, Buddha learned to balance body and mind and to understand the impor-

tance of being present in the moment. These principles later became central to the Buddhist teachings on meditation and the path to enlightenment.

What I find beautiful about yoga is that regardless of faith and belief, there's a practical path to happiness and well-being. There is nothing we need to pray for or hope for; there is something we can do here and now to improve our overall well-being. We can take charge of our own lives regardless of our life situation.

But... there's something more. Something that's hidden. But through yoga, you suddenly notice it. See and hear it.

DMT, or dimethyltryptamine, is a neurotransmitter and a powerful psychoactive substance naturally found in the human body. It has long been the subject of research and speculation in neuroscience and psychology because of its potential role in consciousness and spiritual experiences. While DMT is commonly associated with drugs and hallucinogenic experiences, there are also theories that the body may produce DMT in connection with certain meditative and spiritual states, including yoga.

First and foremost, it's important to note that research on DMT and its role in the body is still limited, and many aspects of its function still need to be fully understood. However, there are some hypotheses and theories about how yoga and medi-tation can affect the production or release of DMT in the body.

One theory is that certain types of meditation and profound spiritual experiences can increase activity in certain parts of the brain, which in turn can stimulate the production of DMT. Some researchers believe that when the brain reaches a state of deep meditation or trance, it may trigger the release of DMT from the pineal gland, a small gland linked to spiritual experiences. There are theories that these effects from yoga can help create the optimal conditions to stimulate the pro-duction of DMT in the body.

Regardless, when we've been practicing yoga for a while, we suddenly see a bright glow at the center of our eyebrows and hear a faint buzzing sound from the top of our heads. Accor-ding to yoga, we activate our chakra system when balan-ced (sattvik). Kundalini Shakti can flow along the spine – a dormant creative force awakened within us. A force we share with the cosmos, and when it reaches our highest chakra, we are one with the universe's intelligence. We become connected and gradually enlightened...

But this is nothing you need to contemplate as a beginner in yoga. It's part of human evolution and happens spontaneous-ly and naturally once you've seated yourself. Just practice your yoga regularly, and the rest will follow.

Best of luck on your journey through life. I hope to see you on my YouTube channel if nothing else.

All the best, and take it slow. Yoga is a marathon, not a 100-meter race. We should be able to engage in yoga until our creator decides to take us home. Soft, calm, and gentle. Observe yourself in the position, your relaxation, breathing, thoughts, and feelings. Then return to the prana in the body – the feeling of warmth and tingling just beneath the skin, again and again… and again. Witness, observe. Witness and observe. Expand your consciousness. Your journey begins.

Mattias (Shreyananda Natha).

Did you like the book? Feel free to follow me on my social media, share and like, tell your friends about the books, and feel free to write an honest review; one or two lines don't matter. All support is precious. Thanks!

On my Facebook page and Instagram, I post exciting news and tips on temporary offers and benefits you can take advantage of. I often also post my yoga routine and other things related to nutrition and health that may be interesting to take part in. So feel free to join them so you don't miss anything interesting:

facebook.com/bhagwanoneofakindbooks

instagram.com/bhagwanoneofakindbooks/

MY BOOKS AND BOOK SERIES

I have two book series that have different audiences. Great Yoga Books – is a series with the most comprehensive fact books on yoga for those who want to explore the subject in depth. Here, you will also find classic yoga books that are rarely translated, such as Patanjali's Yoga Sutras and Hatha Yoga Pradipika. My second series, Yoga Beyond the Poses: The Ultimate Beginner's Guide to Yoga, covers one yoga topic at a time and is extra easy to read with larger text. For those who find it challenging to read extensive books and want a good and broad overview of the subject quickly. Both series are also available as audiobooks.

Teaching Yoga and Meditation Beyond the Poses
– A unique and practical workbook for aspiring yoga teachers who want to teach yoga and meditation beyond the poses.

Teaching Yoga and Meditation Beyond the Poses is a unique and essential resource for new and experienced teachers and a guide for all yoga students interested in refining their skills and knowledge. Teaching Yoga and Meditation is also ideal as a core textbook in yoga teacher training programs.

The book covers fundamental yoga philosophy and history topics, including a historical presentation of classical yoga literature: Yoga Sutras of Patanjali, Bhagavad Gita, etc. Each of the seven major styles of yoga is described, from Hatha yoga, Raja yoga, Tantra yoga, Bhakti yoga, and Kundalini yoga, to knowledge about the chakras, Ayurveda and magic mantras and yantras. The book provides extensive support and tools for teaching integrated and classical yoga (asanas), breathing techniques (pranayama), deep relaxation (Yoga Nidra), and meditation (Ajapa Japa). The book is divided into eight modules with associated knowledge tests and complete yoga and meditation classes.

https://rb.gy/9s6edj

SIGN UP FOR A UNIQUE & FREE CHAIR YOGA CLASS WITH SHREYANANDA NATHA!

DO YOU WANT TO QUICKLY AND EFFECTIVELY LOSE WEIGHT? BECOME MORE FLEXIBLE? IMPROVE YOUR BALANCE? OR FIND PEACE IN LIFE AND RID YOURSELF OF STRESS? NOW YOU HAVE THE CHANCE!

SANKALPA YOGA *IS CLASSICAL YOGA & MEDITATION FOR CHAIRS CREATED BY BEST-SELLING AUTHOR AND YOGA MASTER SHREYANANDA NATHA. IT INCLUDES UNIQUE SERIES OF CHAIR YOGA THAT CAN CHANGE YOUR LIFE HERE AND NOW:*

* **CHAIR YOGA FOR BETTER BALANCE**
* **CHAIR YOGA FOR SOFTER JOINTS**
* **CHAIR YOGA FOR INCREASED STRENGTH**
* **CHAIR YOGA FOR GREATER FLEXIBILITY**
* **CHAIR YOGA FOR IMPROVED FITNESS**
* **CHAIR YOGA FOR WEIGHT LOSS**
* **RELAXATION & MEDITATION**

DURING THE TRIAL CLASS, YOU'LL HAVE THE OPPORTUNITY TO EXPERIENCE WHICH PROGRAM MIGHT SUIT YOU AND THE DEEP-ROOTED EFFECTS OF GENUINE CLASSICAL CHAIR

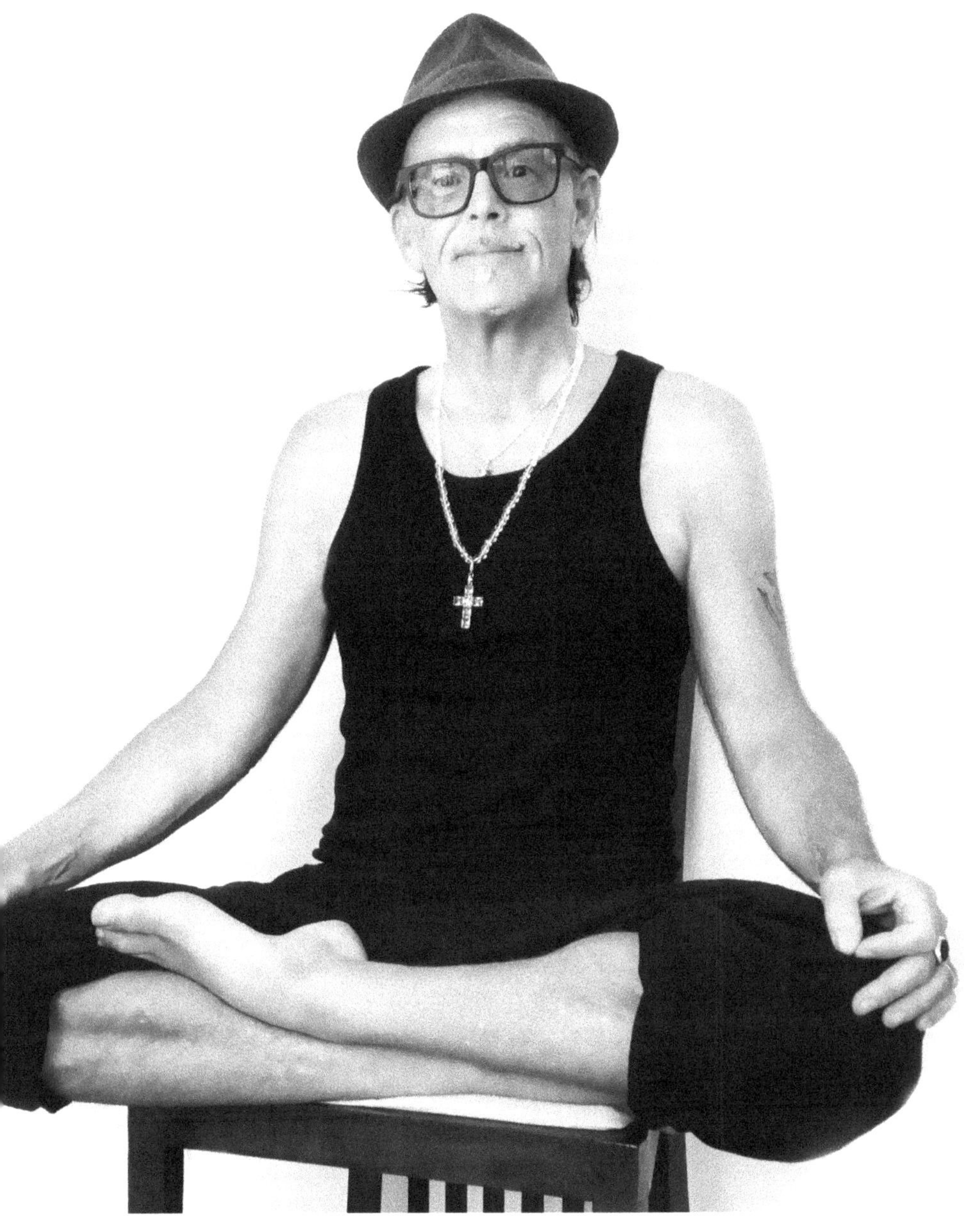

Namo Narayan!

Shreyananda Natha (Mattias)